ALIGNED

THE MODERN MAN'S GUIDE
TO HEALTH, WEALTH & FREEDOM

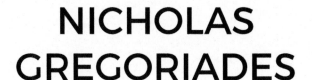

NICHOLAS
GREGORIADES

ALIGNED: A Man's Guide to True Health, Wealth, & Freedom

Copyright Nicholas Gregoriades

Published 1 February 2021 by Fields of Elysium LLC

ISBN: 9798682307371

COACHNICG.COM

DISCLAIMER:

THIS DOCUMENT DETAILS the author's personal experiences with and opinions about health. The advice and strategies contained herein may not be suitable for every situation. This work is sold with the understanding that the author is not a licensed medical or healthcare provider and is not engaged in rendering medical, legal, or other professional advice or services.

The author and publisher are providing this document and its contents on an "as is" basis and make no representations or warranties of any kind with respect to this document or its contents. The author and publisher disclaim all such representations and warranties, including, for example, warranties of merchantability and healthcare for a particular purpose. In addition, the author and publisher do not represent or warrant that the information accessible via this document is accurate, complete, or current.

The statements made about products and services have not been evaluated by the U.S. Food and Drug Administration. They are not intended to diagnose, treat, cure, or prevent any condition or disease. Please consult with your own physician or healthcare specialist regarding the suggestions and recommendations made in this document.

Except as specifically stated in this document, neither the author or publisher, nor any authors, contributors, or other representatives will be liable for damages arising out of or in connection with the use of this document.

This is a comprehensive limitation of liability that applies to all damages of any kind, including (without limitation) compensatory; direct, indirect, or consequential damages; loss of data, income, or profit; loss of or damage to property; and claims of third parties.

You understand that this document is not intended as a substitute for consultation with a licensed healthcare practitioner, such as your physician. Before you begin any healthcare program, or change your lifestyle in any way, you will consult your physician or another licensed healthcare practitioner to ensure that you are in good health and that the examples contained in this document will not harm you.

This document provides content related to physical and/or mental health issues. As such, use of this document implies your acceptance of this disclaimer.

For my mother and father, Gail and Gregory.

"If you must blame your parents for everything that's wrong with you, remember to thank them for everything that's right with you."

TABLE OF CONTENTS

★ ★ ★

INTRODUCTION

—— ★ ★ ★ ——

TAKE A LOOK at where you are in your life: how you spend your time, who you love, how you make money, where you live, what you do for fun.

Now take a deep breath and ask yourself, why am I here?

If you're like most men, you might not have a good answer to that question. But I have an idea of what you *didn't* come here for.

You didn't come here to sit in traffic every day, feeling your energy and passion for life slip away. You didn't come here to lie awake at night, dreading tomorrow.

You didn't come here to spend time with people you don't feel a true connection with. You didn't come here to live in a body that's fat, weak, or unhealthy. You didn't come here to sell your soul doing work you don't find meaningful.

Hell, no. You wanted more than that.

You came here to give your gifts back to the world. You came here for your own unique adventure. You came here to live with passion and joy. You came here to be a creative force in the world.

If you're a man who . . .

✪ knows deep down that he's not fulfilling his potential

✪ has arrived at a point in life where he's thinking, is this all there is to it?

✪ dreams of mastering his health, wealth, and relationships

✪ has achieved a level of success but still feels empty

✪ has lost the spark he used to have for life

✪ wants to reconnect with both his Spirit and Nature

✪ knows he has to make a big change in his life but lacks the confidence required to do so

✪ understands that the human experience is precious and wants to squeeze every last drop out of it

. . . then I've got good news for you: you are destined for that. It's built into who you are.

But before you can achieve it, you must understand and accept that staying as you are will cost you your joy and your health and will ultimately lead to a boring, stale life filled with regret.

But it doesn't have to be that way. With a few small changes to how you live your life, you can be transformed from miserable and unfulfilled to passionate and gratified. You can live the life you want to, and spend every day enjoying the journey.

I know you can accomplish this, no matter how far from it you might feel at this moment. I know because I'm speaking from experience.

Ten years ago, after making some bad decisions, I found myself six thousand miles from home, destitute, out of shape, heartbroken, and alone. People speak of the "dark night of the soul," and believe me when I tell you that period of my life was just about as dark as it gets. I was at my lowest point and I couldn't see a way back into the light.

Then, at my lowest point, I had an epiphany. I realized that I had to stop blaming others for my circumstances—other people, luck, circumstances beyond my control. I took full responsibility for the situation I found myself in. I decided that I had to regain control of my mind, body, and spirit—to completely master myself—if I was going to get out of the hole I was in.

Through a lot of study, deep reflection, and, most importantly, *committed action*, I was able to rebuild my entire life.

Today, at forty-one years old, I'm the happiest and healthiest I've ever been. I have two successful businesses, a fulfilling career, and a huge group of truly incredible friends. I wake up each day excited about life and what it will bring.

I don't tell you this to brag. I just want to show you that it's possible to achieve success, fulfillment, and well-being even if your starting point is as far from those things as you can imagine. As far from those things as I once was, for instance.

On my quest, I learned literally thousands of habits, techniques, strategies, and pieces of wisdom that improved the quality of my human experience and made me a more actualized man. All of these have value, but some have proven *invaluable*.

I've distilled this book down to just twenty essential strategies, those that have been the most transformative and life-changing for both myself and my clients. Most of these tips are very simple, but don't let that dissuade you from implementing them—all are powerful and effective. For the last several years, I've been using what I learned on that journey to help men around the world overcome their self-imposed limitations and become the absolute best versions of themselves.

But before you read any further, I want you to face a certain truth:

This world belongs to those who take action. They get the best of everything. The rest get the dregs.

There's no getting around this fact. There are no shortcuts around it, and you can't fake it. All you can do is accept it and use it to your advantage.

If I had to identify just one thing that has gotten me to where I am today, that has allowed me to live a life that most can only dream of, it's that I am a doer. Sure, I spend huge amounts of time reading, learning, thinking, and planning, but ultimately the fact that I take action is what brings my desires and goals into reality.

That's how I dug myself out of that hole: I took action. Of course, I first had to find the wisdom to act on, but you've got an advantage over me in that department. I've done that part for you by distilling and including the best of what I've learned here in this book.

If you commit to studying these lessons and taking action, I guarantee that in just twenty-eight days you'll be a happier, healthier person, and in six months your life will be almost unrecognizably different.

Notice I said *if*.

At this very moment, right now, you've arrived at a fork in the road of your life. There are two diverging paths before you, each with a very different outcome.

The first path is the most commonly chosen. It looks like this:

You read the rest of this book and find the ideas within inspiring and the potential of a new, better version of yourself appealing. You tell yourself that you're going to implement the information and act on it, but then you get distracted. By anything, really: an errand, a TV show, or some other event. Or you might even make a start and give it the old college try for a few days, but soon find these new habits and mindsets are just too inconvenient, too uncomfortable, or too difficult for you to stick to.

And what happens just down that path? You quickly fall back into your old routines. Nothing changes and you continue living as you always have. This path leads to mediocrity and regret, and it's the one 99.9 percent of the men on this planet, and most of the ones reading this, will take.

The second path is very different and very rarely chosen. It looks like this:

You read the rest of the book, then make a *total commitment* to internalizing and embodying the tools within. This commitment is a promise to yourself, an oath that is bound to both your self-esteem and your integrity.

You don't try. You *decide*. You then take massive, repeated *action*, and you do so *consistently* until the strategies and techniques become habits—until they become a part of *you*.

As I said, very few of the men reading this will choose this second path, but they are the ones who will scale the peaks of life. They are the ones who will have the best health, the most fulfilling careers, and the most satisfying relationships, among other things.

So here you are, at the fork in the road. Down one path is life much as you've lived it so far. You can continue using your current strategies, doing the same stuff you've been trying for years, and hope things will change. Down the other, more difficult path is the potential to achieve the success you deserve.

If you don't want to keep settling for the same old life— if you want to create new possibilities—then you know what you're going to have to do. You have a decision to make.

Which path will you take?

CHOOSE YOUR MISSION

— ★ ★ ★ —

> *There is one quality which one must possess to win, and that is definiteness of purpose, the knowledge of what one wants, and a burning desire to possess it."*
> **—Napoleon Hill**

EVERY MAN HAS to have a mission. Without one, you are vulnerable to forces of distraction and apathy, and you will inevitably drift through your life.

In the Eastern tradition, the male energy represents the active principle on this planet. It is characterized by action, movement, and the ambition to achieve, create, and impose order on the world. A man without a mission—without purpose—is a man missing a fundamental piece of himself.

This can be seen in the typical male–female dating dynamic. You don't need to be rich or good-looking to attract women (although it helps!), but you do need to cultivate a strong sense of purpose. Very few actualized women will tolerate a man who lacks vision for very long.

There's a false belief that your mission has to be something you receive in a flash of insight or are called to do by a higher power. That's why so many of us spend so much time feeling lost—because we are trying to find purpose instead of creating it.

That's right, you can *create* your mission, and it can be anything you want it to be. You don't need anybody's permission to pursue what you want to do with your life, nor do you need anyone else's opinion about what your mission should be. Remember, it's *your* mission—not your dad's mission, not your family's, not society's. Yours.

So how does one go about creating a mission? Fortunately, it can be done after a (relatively) brief period of self-reflection and the use of a few tools. Here are three simple steps that will help you create your own mission, a purpose for living that will drive you on your journey:

1. FIGURE OUT YOUR VALUES

Values motivate our actions by helping us determine what is important to us. Values describe the personal qualities we embody and reflect the beliefs we hold. They are inextricably linked to our aspirations and influence all the decisions we make. Basically, values determine how we move through the world.

If your chosen mission is out of alignment with your values, it's highly unlikely that you'll complete it successfully. And even if you do, it will be deeply unfulfilling and far more difficult than it has to be.

Sometimes, you may have to reconsider your values, especially if they are inherently weak or selfish or they come from a place of fear. If that's the case, this step will require further contemplation, self-reflection, and questioning to figure out how you adopted those values and which ones to replace them with.

2. FIND OUT WHAT LIGHTS YOU UP

I first understood what it meant to be lit up several years ago. I was spending a summer in my hometown of Cape Town, South Africa. I'm an avid kiteboarder, and together with a good friend I spent almost every day of this trip surfing some of the best conditions in the world.

After one particularly phenomenal session, we got out of the water just as the sun was setting. We were both so enlivened, so full of joy and gratitude for what we'd just experienced, that we ran over and hugged each other. It was one of the best moments of my life. I remember thinking, "This is what it means to be *lit up*!"

Being lit up is characterized by an undeniable feeling of connection with the world and yourself. It's a combination of being excited, present, and grateful. It's the state that makes life worth living.

Neither I nor anybody else can tell you what will light you up, as it's a unique and personal thing. But after much experimentation and a strong yearning to reach this state, I can tell you that for me it very often goes hand in hand with:

✪   Spending time with friends

- Spending time in nature

- Participating in a challenging physical activity

- Listening to music

These are a few among many things. Because remember, what lights you up is not only deeply personal, but many activities can be reframed in a way that allows them to light you up.

For example, one of my clients is a financial advisor who had become jaded with his profession. The work we did together allowed him to view what he did in a new light. Instead of seeing it as boring and mechanical, soon he could reframe the work he did for his clients as the invaluable service of being entrusted with their life's savings. This changed everything for him, and soon he was spending each day lit up by something he'd previously lost all passion for.

It shouldn't be too hard to realize what lights you up. What makes you feel inspired? What makes you smile? What makes your whole body tingle and brings tears of joy to your eyes? What is fun? What do you want to be remembered for? What do you spend the currency of your most focused attention on?

3. FORMULATE A MISSION STATEMENT

Once you have figured out what your values are and what lights you up, the last thing you must do is create a mission statement. You'll use this statement as the reference point to guide you forward.

Here's an example from my own life:

- ✪ My values are health, wisdom, self-expression, integrity, and freedom.

- ✪ What lights me up is learning, sharing, being in nature, working out, and connecting with others.

- ✪ My mission on this journey called life is to become the happiest, healthiest, most self-actualized human being I can while helping others do the same, as well as to protect nature and animals from the dark forces that are destroying them.

Notice how my mission follows naturally from the things that are important to me and the things that light me up? It's easy to see that this mission is in total alignment with both of these vital components.

I know every choice I make and circumstance I place myself in must be, at least in the greater scheme of things, favorable to this mission. Otherwise it will lead to weak, indecisive action or failure.

Once you create your mission, one of the most powerful things you will experience is that, almost instantaneously, all tasks related to it require less effort. For example, committing to a challenging ninety-minute workout and a five-mile walk every day doesn't require me to dig deep for motivation because I know they are both aligned with my mission and will help me to achieve it.

Examine your values, find what lights you up, and create a mission that is aligned with both of these. Then commit to it with every fiber of your being.

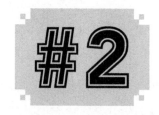

KNOW THAT ALL IS HABIT

— ★ ★ ★ —

People do not decide their futures, they decide their habits and their habits decide their futures."

—F. Matthias Alexander

OF ALL THE lessons I've learned over the last several years, this has been one of the most powerful. If you don't understand and implement this idea, your attempts to use all the other knowledge in this book will probably be ineffective. So pay close attention.

Sometimes we hear things that go straight to our core. It's almost as if the Universe is speaking to us directly through a person or a billboard or a song lyric. That's just what happened to me.

Several years ago, while speaking with my good friend, mentor and eminent philosopher Dr. Khalil Habib, I experienced this phenomenon when he said the words "All is habit." Instantly I knew this particular piece of wisdom was vital. Immediately after the conversation, I spent a long time meditating on this and researching the subject of habits, and what I found convinced me that the impact of habit on our lives is monumental.

You and I can be viewed as simply a collection of habits. Your thoughts are habitual. So are the ways you exercise, dress, and interact with people, and all the other methods by which you move through the world. All are just habits that you have acquired—and, critically, this means they can be eliminated, changed, replaced, improved, or embraced.

But this is key: doing so requires you to go through an initial period of discipline and may involve some difficulty or discomfort. This is just the price you have to pay to gain (or lose) a habit and reap the reward. There is no other way. Internalize that fact and make peace with it.

The great news, though, is that once you make it through this initially challenging period, the habit takes over and does most of the work for you.

HABIT FORMATION

So, just how does someone alter their habits? I've discovered a few steps that can help you find the initial discipline to pick up or lose a habit:

1. Place the habits you want to create/break into the context of your values and mission statement.

2. Track your habit formation progress religiously. One of the sayings I live my life by is "That which is measured improves." Very few positive things come with

being attached to your smartphone constantly, but one of them is that you can use it as a tool to track and monitor your habits.

3. Ask yourself during moments of struggle, what are the consequences if I don't do this? This question can be effective because potential negative outcomes are sometimes more motivating than positive ones.

Here's an example from my own life. I recently decided to pick up the habit of doing twenty minutes of light stretching and mobility work first thing after waking up. I noticed that when I do this, everything flows more smoothly, and I am more physically relaxed and mentally calm for the rest of the day.

Now, if I look at this habit in relation to my values (health) and my mission statement (become the healthiest human being I can be), it's an absolute no-brainer. That did wonders for my motivation early in the morning, especially during the first few weeks.

After each mobility session, I grabbed my smartphone and used a habit-tracking app to record the session. Being able to see my success inspired me to strive for further success.

But these two tips still didn't make it easy to change my habits every time. Whenever I hesitated or wavered in my commitment to my mobility routine, I reminded myself that this habit will have such a huge impact in helping me complete my mission. I reflected on the fact that if I don't create this positive habit, I will continue to lose mobility as I age, which will massively compromise my health and quality of life.

It only took a few weeks of stretching each morning before it became automatic, and after several months, it actually became harder to skip it than to do it. The habit had taken over—no more willpower required.

Now I don't need to think about doing it each morning; it just gets done. I have freed up mental energy and gained a practice that moves me closer to the person I want to be, all after just a few weeks of disciplined action.

That's a small example. But you can train yourself into (or out of) just about any habit. Charles Duhigg explains the psychology and science behind habits exceptionally well in *The Power of Habit*. I strongly suggest you get this book and read it as if your life depends on it . . . because it does.

Once you eliminate the habits that are holding you back and create the positive ones that will propel you forward (the most important of which are outlined throughout this guide), your life will begin to change in dramatic fashion.

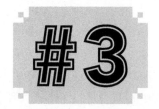

MEDITATE EVERY DAY

— ★ ★ ★ —

> *Meditation will not carry you to another world, but it will reveal the most profound and awesome dimensions of the world in which you already live."*
>
> **—Zen Master Hsing Yun**

IF YOU CAME to me with a briefcase containing ten million dollars and said it was mine on the condition that I quit meditating for the rest of my life, I'd turn you down in a heartbeat.

When I became aware that we are more than just physical beings and that there is more to reality than meets the eye, I embarked on a journey to learn as much as possible about these esoteric aspects of the human experience. I read every book I could get my hands on and went down some very deep rabbit holes.

Over the course of this journey, I discovered two things that stood out. First, there is a huge amount of what I call "spiritual garbage" in the world—so many empty promises, so much woo-woo crap being sold and marketed to the naive and desperate.

I consider myself extremely open-minded, but I'm also inherently skeptical. My training in the functional martial art of jiu jitsu really helped keep me grounded. Unlike many of the traditional martial arts, which make huge claims and bold promises, in jiu jitsu, something either works or it doesn't. No metaphysical explanation necessary, just what you see with your own eyes.

So whenever I engage in any philosophical or spiritual endeavor, at the root of my engagement is always that same question: Does this work? Does it make my life noticeably better? Does it make me more successful? Does it improve my experience as I move through the world? As Bruce Lee said, "Absorb what is useful, reject what is useless."

I have tried many, many supposedly spiritual things and evaluated them using this same test. Mediation and plant medicine were the only two things I encountered that passed the test, and meditation in particular offered something I've never experienced anywhere else. In fact, meditation is one of the very few genuine keys to the realm of Spirit.

THE BENEFITS OF MEDITATION

Meditating and becoming aware of your breathing patterns are some of the most important habits you will ever form, and they will pay dividends in all areas of your life. I wrote an article several years ago called "Life Tastes Better with Meditation," which comes the closest to describing the far-reaching effects it has had on my life. It just makes everything better. Food, sex, nature—all are enhanced by this extraordinary practice.

So even if exploring the esoteric concepts is not your thing, then just forget the spiritual aspect of the process and focus on the documented mental and physical benefits. It is beyond debate that regular meditation will make you calmer, happier, and more productive. It will also improve your creativity. It lowers blood pressure, reduces stress and anxiety, and improves the quality of your sleep.

There are several ways it does these things. The first is by acting as an antidote to the stimulation-obsessed modern world. If you're over thirty years old, you're old enough to remember that life didn't always contain a constant barrage of smartphone notifications and text messages. The only screens we used to engage with were televisions—and even then only for a couple of hours each day.

The fact is that modern life has trained us to concentrate only in short bursts and has caused our brains to become addicted to constant dopamine spikes. Neither of these is conducive to a calm, healthy mind.

Meditation can immunize you against this. During meditation practice, you eliminate external stimuli and redirect your focus onto a single point. If you do this regularly, it begins to improve your attention span and wean you off the constant need for novelty (compulsively checking your phone, playing a video game, engaging in gossip, etc.). Without these kinds of superficial distractions, you can then use your undivided mental resources to create, work, or build a better life for yourself.

Another powerful benefit of regular meditation is a stronger connection between you and your breath. Your breath is your primary interface with life itself, and it plays a huge role in the quality of your life. It's said that you can go without food for a few weeks and without water for a few days, but without air for only a few minutes.

As I always teach my jiu jitsu students: Your breath is inextricably connected to your performance on the mat. If you are not breathing correctly, you won't be able to fight effectively.

But it goes far beyond the martial arts mat. We breathe throughout our lives, and the quality of our breathing patterns is directly proportional to the quality of our awareness. If our breathing is slow, deep, and even, our minds are calm and non-reactive. If we breathe rapidly or shallowly, we become agitated and anxious and emotionally labile.

Years of stress and poor posture have ruined the breathing patterns of many people. Instead of deep, slow, even breaths, we breathe high in our chests and sometimes even forget to breathe. Meditation reverses these patterns and allows us to create a strong awareness of how the breath moves into and out of our bodies.

Here's an example of the immediate benefits of meditation practice:

John's boss comes into his office, closes the door behind him, and says, "We need to talk." John assumes something is wrong and immediately his body releases a cascade of stress hormones. He starts to tense up. This tension then causes his breathing to become shallow, which causes his awareness to contract—this is characterized by racing thoughts or fixation. All he can think about is the potential humiliation of being reprimanded or fear of being fired.

If John had been meditating regularly, he would have remained better connected to his breath. This would have allowed him to stay present, consider all options and scenarios in his mind, and respond in the most advantageous manner. The release of stress hormones would have been minimal, and he would have returned to a steady state far more quickly.

A BASIC SEATED MEDITATION

All right, so meditation is a good habit to pick up (for example, using the habit formation tips in the previous chapter). How exactly is one to do that? There are many versions of meditation, each with their particular set of methods and benefits. In my experience, the most powerful of all of these is the basic seated meditation.

The purpose of this style of meditation is to quiet the chattering of the mind by bringing your awareness to a single point of focus through concentration. Best of all, you can perform it anywhere without any expensive tools, though I recommend a quiet place, an app called Insight Timer, and whatever cushions or mats will help you sit comfortably.

Here is a brief guide to performing it properly:

- ✪ Choose and commit to a regular time each day when you will not be disturbed. Early morning or late night works best.

- ✪ Create a quiet, dark place where you will not be disturbed.

- ✪ Sit in whatever position is comfortable for you.

✪ Open the Insight Timer app on your phone and create a preset for nine minutes. Include interval bells at the three- and six-minute marks. (I suggest you make the start, end, and interval bells all different sounds.)

✪ Put your phone on airplane mode and start the timer.

✪ At the start bell: Close your eyes and scan your body mentally from head to toe. Try to consciously relax any tense areas you discover, particularly in the face, jaw, and neck. After that, just allow your mind to wander.

✪ At the first interval bell: bring your awareness to the sensation (primary) and sound (secondary) of your breath entering and exiting your nostrils.

✪ Whenever you catch yourself becoming distracted or lost in thought, bring your awareness back to your breath for a full ten count. Then stay focused on your breathing without the count.

✪ If you become distracted again, just repeat the count. Continue until the ending bell.

Each week add three minutes to the timer. So during week two, the total time will be twelve minutes, with interval bells at the four- and eight-minute marks, and week three will increase by another three total minutes.

Note: For this to be effective, you need to do it for at least 28 consecutive days.

You cannot judge whether meditation is working for you until you've done it consistently. Make a deal with yourself that you're going to do it for twenty-eight days straight, and set up a way to count each day. If you miss a day, start the count from one again. Keep going until you are doing regular thirty-minute sessions.

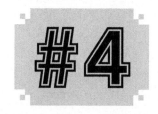

COMMIT TO EXCELLENCE

———— ★ ★ ★ ————

"*Excellence is doing ordinary things extraordinarily well.*"

—John W. Gardener

ASIDE FROM YOUR individual mission, odds are good you want what most people do: professional success, material goods, the respect of your peers and loved ones. Unfortunately, there are nearly eight billion people on this planet, and they all want pretty much the same things you do. That means competition is immense. If your work and output are anything less than excellent, you have no chance.

That's one of the things I love about living in America, where this is most evident. It forces me to raise my game because there's no space in this society for average. Everyone needs to be smart and work hard or they get left behind.

Now I know the gulf between what you consider excellent and what you are currently capable of can seem overwhelming. Trust me, I've been there. But the solution is the Japanese idea of *kaizen* — that small but consistent improvements lead to massive growth over time. If you commit to getting just 1 percent better each day at anything, in a year you'll be over three times better than you were before.

This is closely related to another idea that, when internalized and acted on, will completely revolutionize your life:

Be so good they can't ignore you.

Dedication to excellence is the cure for almost all career and financial troubles. When you do great work, create great products, or give great service, money and career advancement will come naturally as a byproduct.

When I set out to build my jiu jitsu business, I had no name in the industry. The world of functional martial arts puts a lot of stock in your professional record as a fighter. Unless you're a world champion or one of the best competitors globally, it's very difficult to get noticed.

Even though I was a world-class fighter, I never made it into the upper echelons. So I directed my focus on becoming such a good teacher that they couldn't ignore me. I read books on pedagogy, practiced my presentation, prepared my classes thoroughly, and devoted myself to constant improvement. After time, diligent practice, and a lot of effort, I became a true master of my craft.

And as soon as I did, the word about me spread. Soon I was in demand and teaching around the world.

"How you do one thing is how you do everything."

If you approach the small things in life with a total, un-wavering commitment to excellence, then it's almost certain you'll do the same for the big, important things.

To use another example from my own life, I do every-thing—the way I walk, breathe, communicate, pay for some-thing in a store, fold the towels before I put them away—with intense focus and attention to detail. When you do even small tasks with this kind of conscious intention, excellence soon be-comes a habit. That's why I make such an effort to keep order around me, especially in my home.

After twenty years as a professional jiu jitsu teacher, the biggest lesson I have learned is that there's always a better way to do something. In jiu jitsu, being sloppy or lazy with your techniques or movements will always cost you. You don't just grab your opponent's arm and yank on it—instead, you use a precise, economical movement, and you use it with intention.

It's the same in life as a whole. This kind of awareness, and the ability to put it into action daily, are key factors that not only separate world-class athletes from the rest, but also set apart self-actualized and successful human beings.

MASTER YOUR PHYSICALITY

——— ★ ★ ★ ———

No man has the right to be an amateur in the matter of physical training. It is a shame for a man to grow old without seeing the beauty and strength of which his body is capable."

—Socrates

MEN WHO ARE in shape exude a completely different energy compared to those who don't. They have better posture and a more confident presence, and they move through the world more assertively. We are physical beings, so it's imperative that you master the physical vehicle you are using to navigate this life.

It is my opinion that the two most important physical practices you can engage in to maximize your health and longevity are mobility work and resistance training.

As you age, both of these change from "important" to "vital." Two primary predictors of quality of life as we age are strength and mobility. The stronger you are, the less pronounced degeneration will be as you age. Keep in mind that a man's muscle mass decreases by 1 percent per year after the age of thirty. That might not sound like much, but trust me when I tell you that by the time you're forty, if you've lost 10 percent of the muscle you had at thirty, you will feel it big time.

Resistance training has been said to be "as close to the fountain of youth as a man can get." This is because it offers the safest, most reliable, and most easily measurable way to negate the aforementioned two hallmarks of physical decline. It also raises the metabolic rate in both the short term and the long term, and it increases balance and muscle control. So, in short, make sure you're lifting heavy things at least twice a week. This can include weights or kettlebells, but it can also be your own body weight.

Mobility is just as important as resistance training. One of the most powerful quotes I've ever heard is: "You're only as old as your joints." If you're twenty-five and have a creaky, stiff body, you're effectively old, but a seventy-year-old with mobile, healthy joints is as fit as a young person. If you're doing resistance training, it's especially important to focus on your mobility to avoid creating imbalances in your musculoskeletal system.

Finally, a good workout not only benefits your physique but has a huge positive impact on your mental health. Whenever I'm feeling less than my best or find negativity creeping in, a solid workout is my first countermeasure because it almost always turns things around. This is why I insist that everyone I work with dedicates themselves to some form of exercise three to four times per week. It's the foundation for everything else.

WHICH FORMS OF EXERCISE ARE THE BEST?

One of the biggest blessings to come out of my previous career as a professional martial artist is advanced knowledge about the most effective ways of working out.

Functional martial arts (MMA, boxing, wrestling, judo, BJJ, grappling, Muay Thai) require a physique that is more than just strong—it needs to be flexible, coordinated, and adaptive. So when I became a competitive martial artist, I had to find the best conditioning routines possible. If something was ineffective, I didn't have the time or energy to waste on it, and if it was effective, I milked it for all it was worth.

I started with classic bodybuilding protocols, using dumbbells, barbells, and traditional resistance-training machines. These were excellent for increasing muscle mass and building a decent level of strength, but were lacking in other areas.

After a few years, I decided to take a hiatus from all forms of resistance training except those that employed my own body weight. I began to focus exclusively on gymnastic and calisthenic movements. After this change I noticed significant improvements in my mobility and muscular endurance, but I missed the ability to adjust the resistance incrementally. I also found that except for pull-ups, very few options were available for pulling-type movements. There had to be a form of exercise that could do it all.

During a trip to Australia around the time the CrossFit and "functional training" movements were becoming popular, I attended a kettlebell training course. After spending several weeks experimenting with and learning about these interesting tools, I was struck by how perfectly they were suited to conditioning for the combat sports in which I was involved. They provided strength and power without stiffness, improved coordination, and allowed me to practice the all-important pulling exercises so vital for good jiu jitsu performance. Best of all, because of their versatility and compact size, it finally became possible to pursue total fitness in a home gym.

Although I believe dumbbell and barbell training (and to a much lesser extent, resistance machines) have their place in a man's training regimen, I find the combination of body weight exercises and kettlebell lifts ideal for most. All you need is a little space at home and a couple of kettlebells.

Other excellent forms of exercise feature elements of resistance training, of course. Rock climbing, "flow" styles of yoga, and functional martial arts like boxing, wrestling, jiu jitsu, and Muay Thai are examples.

Keep in mind the following guidelines when planning your own exercise regimen.

Whatever you strengthen you must stretch, and whatever you stretch you must strengthen.

Neglecting either is a recipe for injury. I suggest supplementing your resistance training sessions with weekly yoga classes or at the very least doing ten to fifteen minutes of stretching at the end of your workout. Posture is everything. For most of us, the major issue is tight hip flexors and tight pectorals. Also, a forward head position can become an issue if you sit at a desk for long periods. Few things cause the amount of physical degeneration that can come from this type of long-term, stationary activity day after day.

Consistency beats intensity.

After reading something inspirational (like this book), most of us tend to dive into a super-challenging six-days-a-week program. This almost always leads to burnout and abandonment of the exercise habit. It's far better to work out two to three times per week every week of the year than to do five or more sessions a week and flame out after a month.

Exercise should leave you feeling energized, not exhausted.

Don't buy into the mentality that you need to be working so hard that you puke, or that pain is a good sign. Yes, there is truth in the adage "If exercise is easy to do, it's hard to benefit from, and if it's hard to do, it's easy to benefit from." But there's a difference between challenging and destructive.

Recovery is essential.

The primary indicator of whether you are ready to exercise should be how you feel. If you are fresh and energetic, go for it. If you are still sore and thoroughly drained from a previous workout, you should rest that day or do some less strenuous activity like yoga or walking. Having said that, don't mistake physical exhaustion for laziness or lack of discipline. If you're honest with yourself, you'll know the difference.

CREATE MORE THAN YOU CONSUME

★ ★ ★

> "To practice any art, no matter how well or badly, is a way to make your soul grow. So do it."
>
> **—Kurt Vonnegut**

A STORY I'M fond of relating is about a man who did a ceremony with the incredibly powerful psychedelic iboga. The journey took him right down to the building blocks of his psyche—it showed him all the formative memories of his childhood that ultimately shaped the man he became. When he recounted this truly powerful experience, the thing he found most notable (and terrifying) was just how much advertising there was at that base level of his mind.

Your whole life, you've been trained to be a consumer. It probably started with Saturday morning cartoons and then progressed to comics, books, video games, music, television, etc. You were trained to consume not only content, but goods. One of the most pervasive messages in our society is that getting something will make you more content or give you peace of mind.

There is nothing wrong with experiencing and enjoying the content of others, or with having nice things. But no matter their quality, I can assure you that they will not bring you the same level of fulfillment as the act of creating things yourself.

As a human being, you come with an innate creative impulse, and if that impulse is not expressed in a healthy way, you will never feel fulfilled. That's one of the reasons a guy with a banking job can have a seven-figure salary and all the toys in the world and still feel miserable.

I first developed an understanding of this concept while watching an interview with Brené Brown, author of *The Gifts of Imperfection*. Brown explained that the creative impulse within human beings is always there, and if it is not followed or engaged with, it will manifest in negative and toxic ways. It sounds a little out there, but my own experience and observation of the experiences of my clients and others assures me there's some truth to it.

In fact, your own experience should bear this out as well. Ever notice how unsatisfied you feel after spending several hours surfing the internet, watching TV, or playing a video game? Or how the moment after you purchase something, you are often accompanied by a feeling of emptiness?

But creating is not just more fulfilling than consuming. When harnessed properly, it's also more likely to help you achieve your goals. Creation is closely aligned with production, and as MJ De Marco explains in his incredible book *Unscripted*, producers (creators) are the ones who win the greatest prizes in our society. Those who create things that improve the quality of the human experience—through amazing products, services, or art—get the biggest rewards.

PLAY MORE

Very closely related to the importance of creativity is play. When was the last time you just played without any end goal in mind? That's one of the main reasons people get old quickly: they become overly serious. Everything becomes so "important." A predominant belief of our culture is that work and suffering are noble, but play and fun are infantile.

In my popular *Spirit of Jiu Jitsu* video, I discuss the concept of *lila*, which is Sanskrit for "divine playfulness." Hinduism holds the perspective that our world and everything in creation is the Universe expressing itself through play. I don't know if that's true in any literal sense, but it resonates with me.

Even work can be reframed as play. That's one of the reasons doing what you love can bring you great success: because things you love usually involve playing or creating, or a combination of both. And everyone loves playing and creating.

Learning is also closely aligned with this concept. Your brain is a learning machine, and it thrives on developing new skills and abilities. The next time you just want to slump in front of the television, consider instead learning to draw, mastering a new language, or taking up a musical instrument. These might seem like daunting prospects, but remember, "starting is half done." Just the act of beginning something— that first step of watching an instructional video or opening a book or putting pen to paper—means you are far more likely to continue it to completion. Don't overthink it. Just take that first step, then follow the steps necessary to create the habit.

You might be thinking, but learning and studying involve consuming content! And yes, that's true. But don't confuse watching or reading for study purposes with mindless consumption. For some reason I can't quite figure out, consuming with the intention of learning a skill isn't quite the same. Perhaps it's because as you read with intention, you are creating new wisdom within yourself.

DROP THE PORN

★ ★ ★

> *Feed your mind with the good, the clean, the pure, the powerful, and the positive."*
>
> **—Zig Ziglar**

AROUND THE SAME time that I began to meditate regularly, I began to develop greatly increased self-awareness. Specifically, I became hyper-aware of the way people, places, and things affected my energy and the way I felt. In particular, I started to notice that each time I engaged with porn, I felt several negative effects. Not only did I feel literally and figuratively drained, but I noticed that it was having detrimental effects on my mood and ability to concentrate. More importantly, I began to notice a deep instinct that it wasn't good for me.

Then I watched the 2013 film *Don Jon*. It follows the story of a guy who develops unrealistic expectations from watching porn, and this cripples his ability to have a healthy relationship. Eventually he overcomes his addiction and finds happiness and real intimacy with his potential true love. I really identified with the film and saw aspects of my own experience reflected in it.

I'd like to note that the views I hold on this subject do not come from a religious or puritanical place. I myself used porn on occasion for most of my twenties and early thirties, and I make no judgments about anyone who still does so. After doing a lot of research on the mental and physical effects of pornography, however, I arrived at the perspective that it is toxic to the mind, the body, and the soul, and it has no place in the life of a man who is striving to be the best version of himself.

THE DARK SIDE

I want you to imagine a spectrum of human experience. On one end are the things most of us intrinsically regard as positive—composure, contentment, clarity, self-mastery, health. On the other end are the attributes and states of mind that we view with disdain and seek to avoid—discontent, impatience, impulsiveness, greed, confusion. To me, almost any action or experience can be located somewhere on this spectrum, and it's quite obvious where porn falls.

Porn hijacks the circuitry of your brain and causes you to become addicted to sexual novelty and to the subsequent dopamine spikes released by viewing it. Unfortunately, you also become very quickly desensitized to this novelty and require more unusual or extreme stimulus, which is usually accompanied by increasing levels of depravity.

Porn feeds the urge for instant gratification and fuels greed and excess. In this way, it is destructive to the soul.

A close friend of mine once worked with someone—let's call him Steve—who got a job with one of the big porn sites. Steve's role was to filter out the submitted videos for anything illegal or too extreme. Basically, he watched porn all day and got paid for it. Sounds pretty sweet, right? Well, after a few months, when my friend saw Steve again, he was shocked at the deterioration in his physical and psychological state. My friend said, "All I kept thinking was that he reminded me of Gollum from *Lord of the Rings*—sickly and anxious. He couldn't even look me in the eye anymore."

Now sure, that's completely anecdotal, but stories like this are not rare. I saw firsthand how porn destroyed the relationship between one of my best friends and his girlfriend. His casual interaction with it very quickly became a habit he couldn't break, and it led to unrealistic expectations. This put a huge amount of pressure on their physical relationship and ultimately tore them apart.

Everything good, healthy, and wholesome in life has a shadow version that promises the same outcome. The example I often cite on my podcast is eating. At the highest level, eating is a community experience that is done to nourish the body. Think of sitting down with your family to leisurely enjoy a home-cooked meal made with love and quality ingredients. The shadow version of this is grabbing some low-grade takeout and shoveling it down in a stressed state while thinking about work or other matters. They are both considered eating, but they are two very different things. One is a shadow of the other.

Porn is the shadow of a healthy, loving sexual relationship between a man and his partner.

WHY GIVE IT UP?

It can seem like you're getting something for free with porn, but I can assure you that you're not. Porn trains you to associate sex and your sexual energy with fantasy as opposed to reality. Sex, like everything else, is best when you're fully present. You cannot genuinely connect with someone else if you are not present, let alone when you *are* in a sexual context.

If you're already in a relationship and you use porn, it's a safe bet that your relationship is not going nearly as well as it could be. Even if you're not cheating in the traditional sense, you're still diverting your sexual energy in a different direction.

If you're in a relationship, eliminating porn from your life will improve it. If you're single, it will make you more attractive to potential partners because you'll have a completely different energy when you interact with them. You will be far less likely to look at them as mere sex objects and instead be able to create a genuine connection, which is the foundation of all great relationships, including sexual ones.

Now, I get it. I'm a man, and I have a high sex drive. I know giving up porn isn't easy, especially if you're single. The world we live in shoves sex in our faces so often, it's impossible not to be drawn to it. My experience has been that the answer to this problem is transmutation and redirection. You must rechannel that energy into your work and your mission or, at the very least, save it for real-life physical intimacy.

Besides eliminating porn from your life, you might consider engaging in a program designed to help you master your sexual energy. Many of these are available online.

If you make the committed decision to drop the porn, you will reap multiple rewards that far exceed the shallow, damaging thing you've given up.

#8

MINIMIZE YOUR ALCOHOL USE

★ ★ ★

"*Almost anything can be preserved in alcohol, except health, happiness, and money.*"

—**Mary Wilson Little**

ALCOHOL IS RESPONSIBLE for more failed relationships, more physical violence, more illness and death, and more unfulfilled dreams than any other substance in the history of civilization.

Here's the bottom line: if you're having more than a couple of units of alcohol per week, you're compromising your health and limiting your potential in several areas of your life.

Now there's probably a part of you that will try to rationalize these facts away. "But I need it to socialize!" "It's boring being out with my friends when I haven't had a few drinks." "It helps me relax." Frankly, that's all bullshit.

First, if you can't relax around people without having a drink, that's indicative of some social anxiety issues that you need to face like a man instead of numbing them away with alcohol.

And second, if your friends pressure you to drink when you're around them, it's because they are being reminded of their own inability to function in a social setting without a crutch, and they are trying (consciously or not) to pull you back down to their level. If you speak honestly with them about why you're not drinking and they still can't handle it, then I suggest you start looking for some better friends.

One of my clients didn't believe me about how much alcohol was compromising all the parts of his life until I got him to stay off it for a while. After just a few days, his head started to clear and he began to sleep better. His mood became more optimistic, and his days became characterized by clarity and purpose for the first time in years.

If you drink regularly, you have probably forgotten what it feels like to have your default, sober state be a good one. You don't know what it's like to have a sharp, clear mind and a truly healthy, strong body. How can you when you're effectively poisoning yourself several times per week?

Recently a friend related that he wanted to save up money for a new car. His new budgeting strategy included drinking at home before going out because it was cheaper than purchasing alcohol at the bar. I literally couldn't believe what I was hearing. To be so dependent on a drug that you're unable to socialize without it is a clear sign that something is wrong in your life.

Do not accept this as normal just because almost everybody else does it. It's not normal.

A BETTER ROAD

Don't you want to be the kind of person who doesn't require a crutch to feel good, the kind of person who can be authentic and social without using a drug to change his state first? Make no mistake, alcohol is a drug, and it's in a specific class called "depressants." Yes, depressants usually have the effect of lowering your mood, but physiologically they impair and slow the activity of the brain and nervous system. That's why it feels "good" to have a couple of drinks—because you spend most of your waking life so wired from stress and overstimulation that anything that slows you down brings immediate relief.

But do you know what can do that on a permanent basis, for free, without negative side effects? Meditation. In some ways, as porn is the shadow version of a loving sexual relationship that promises the same benefits but delivers nothing but emptiness, alcohol is used as a shadow version of meditation.

Having said that, alcohol is still a ubiquitous part of the human experience. Even though total abstinence is a valid route that is infinitely healthier than regular consumption, I think the best alternative is to have an extremely disciplined and moderated approach. For example, having one to two drinks very infrequently can be a healthy choice.

Personally, I have a couple of beers a month, primarily because I want to shift my state from its default a little and get a new perspective. But even after two beers, I always feel off my game the next day: not quite as sharp, not quite as motivated. And I don't want to be anything but my best if I can help it.

If you still have doubts, try doing a simple cost–benefit analysis. Ask yourself: is the fun you have while drunk worth the way you feel the next day? And is it worth compromising all the healthy habits and routines you are building and have built?

For me, the answer is clear. I think it will be to you, too.

FAST INTERMITTENTLY

— ★ ★ ★ —

> "Start the practice of self-control with some penance; begin with fasting."
>
> **—Mahavira**

THERE ARE HUNDREDS of interesting and persuasive theories on diet and nutrition, but as is often the case, the real world gives us far more applicable wisdom. I saw one of my first examples of this principle when I was still a teenager.

I had just begun studying physical culture and nutrition, and I was consuming a huge amount of information on these topics. I was explaining to a friend's father that, according to studies I'd been reading, certain people were genetically pre-destined to be fat regardless of the quality or quantity of what they ate. He listened patiently and then said, "That's total bullshit. If that's the case, how come there are no fat people in concentration camps?"

Now, I get that it may be a very crude line of thinking, but I couldn't answer him. And I realized there was some truth to what he said.

If you're honest with yourself, and you're committed to living up to your peak potential, you cannot allow yourself to be overweight. I'm not saying you need to be ripped and have an eight-pack. But unless you have an illness or disease that affects your ability to stay in shape, being overweight sends a couple of very clear messages to the world: you don't take pride in your appearance, and you lack discipline.

A SIMPLE SOLUTION

One of my favorite expressions, one I live my life by, is "A complex problem always requires a simple solution." And the fact is, weight loss and nutrition in the modern age have become unnecessarily complex problems.

There are so many systems, diets, and exercise programs on the market, most with conflicting advice. It can be so overwhelming that many people never take steps to improve their body composition because they become paralyzed by the complexity of it all.

Every few years, a new craze uses carefully selected studies and highly massaged statistics to try to convince us that omitting a certain food group or adding a supplement—or lifting weights as fast as you can until you vomit—will deliver your ideal weight and athletic physique. At the time of writing this, we're in the "Keto and CrossFit" phase, albeit toward the end of it.

But remember, anyone who tells you that their way is the only or best method of achieving something is either untruthful or ignorant. We are all individuals, and there are many paths each of us may take. Once again, your own experience can be your guide:

Have you noticed that for every single diet rule, there are countless people who disprove it? The keto crew says carbs and sugar make you fat. But one of my best friends eats a ton of sugar and is lean and healthy. The low-fat tribe says fat is the enemy and causes obesity and heart disease. But I know a guy in his eighties who looks great for his age and eats bacon and eggs almost every single day of his life. If you dig deep enough into any dietary theory, you can find countless exceptions that call it into question.

In my own fitness quest, I have used myself as a guinea pig for most of the fad diets out there. I have been a vegan or a vegetarian, eaten nothing but meat for six weeks, and on and on. In all that time, I found exactly one thing that works.

THE BIG SECRET

I want to share with you the biggest diet secret of all time. I had to dive to the bottom of the Mariana Trench and dig it out of a treasure chest in a sunken pirate ship. It's been confirmed clinically effective by a team of scientists from MIT, and I have it on good authority that nine out of ten Instagram fitness models swear by it. Naturally, given what I said above, this is not the only way to get fit, and nothing is guaranteed without the discipline and dedication to stick to it, but in my experience, this secret works in a way other fad diets don't.

Are you ready? Here it goes:

Your body requires a certain amount of fuel for energy. If you consume more of that fuel than your body needs, it will store the excess in the form of fat. To get rid of this fat, you need to either burn more energy than you consume, or consume less than you burn.

That's it. That's the absolute last diet secret you'll ever need. But I can't package that and turn it into a best-selling program or book—nobody can. That's why this straightforward concept is not commonly held up as the ultimate answer by diet gurus in mainstream media. It's too simple, and not enough money can be made off of it. Yet it's undeniable that most humans in the modern world eat far too much and far too often, and this is why we get fat.

That's what I love about the **intermittent fasting protocol**—it's so incredibly simple and straightforward. There is no food group to restrict, no weekly meal plan, and no shakes to mix. There is only one rule to adhere to: you limit your eating window to a certain amount of time per day. It doesn't really even matter that much what you eat (within reason), as long as you stick to that one simple rule.

There are several different fasting protocols, but the one I've had the most success with is 18:6. This means you have an eighteen-hour stretch of fasting and a six-hour window in which you can eat each day. Your lifestyle and commitments dictate which span of six hours you choose to eat in, but for me, eating between 12:00 p.m. and 6:00 p.m. has been very effective. I also do this only on weekdays and then relax a bit on the weekends. If you have a family, make sure you align your eating window with family mealtimes.

Keep in mind that although it will probably be challenging for the first couple of days, the body adapts very quickly. Soon you'll wonder how you used to eat so often. If it's too difficult initially, start with a 16:8 fast three days per week, then gradually increase the frequency and duration of your fast.

How does it work, though? When you practice intermittent fasting, there are long stretches when your stomach has nothing in it, so it begins to shrink and your appetite naturally decreases. As a result, you take in fewer calories, which means your body starts running at a caloric deficit and begins using existing fat stores for energy.

Keep in mind that if you fast, there is the possibility of muscle wastage. Your body will catabolize both fat and muscle when operating at a caloric deficit. And here's where another wonderful benefit of resistance training comes into play. If you're doing frequent resistance training, when it comes time to choose to burn fat or muscle, the body is much more likely to choose fat.

There are several other benefits to fasting. Because so much energy is used in the digestive process, most people find they have much more energy when they adopt this way of eating. Freeing up this energy allows it to be used for more creative and productive endeavors. It also saves time that was previously spent on cooking, preparing, and seeking out food.

FASTING FOR THE MIND

Additionally, fasting has some powerful psychological and spiritual benefits. At the root of many of our choices is the fear of hunger. On a subconscious level, many of us stay in jobs we hate or make huge life decisions based solely on the financial implications. The reason for this is because deep down, in our lizard brains, we're afraid of going hungry. The thing is, when you've gotten used to the feeling of being hungry and realize that not only is it not that bad, but it also comes with several benefits, that fear loses a lot of the power it once had.

It's *good* to feel hungry sometimes. It sharpens all of the senses and causes a feeling of lightness in the body. Your digestive system is finally allowed to take a much-needed break. I've also found it engenders a hunger for life; when I fast, the docile, placated state of being that emerges after I consume a big meal is a less frequent occurrence.

After just two weeks of intermittent fasting, a close friend of mine said, "I'm not a slave to food anymore." I can't help but agree with him. He verbalized something I'd been feeling ever since I began the practice.

When I do eat, I don't deprive myself or feel guilty about anything I consume. But I also don't gorge myself or eat much low-quality, overly processed food. The result is a healthier me on every level.

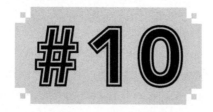

REALIZE IT'S NOT ABOUT THE MONEY

— ★ ★ ★ —

> *Making money isn't hard in itself. What's hard is to earn it doing something worth devoting one's life to."*
> **—Carlos Ruiz Zafón**

IF YOU'RE READING this, a large part of your life has been influenced by money. Think of how many choices in your life have been either directly or indirectly affected by money. If you trace them back, the answer is probably close to 90 percent, especially in your adult life.

I enjoy money just as much as the next guy, if not more. But it's not a focus of my life anymore. I no longer ask, how much money will this make me? Instead I ask, how much service can I provide here? How much fun will this be? How aligned is this with my mission? Those are the questions that make a real difference.

Personal development guru Steve Pavlina shared an observation in his blog about the show *Star Trek* that really allowed me to view money in a new light. Here's an excerpt from the article:

Each character is clear about his/her purpose in life. Each one works within the area of overlap between passion, expertise, need, and purpose. They don't work for money but rather for personal fulfillment. There is some type of economy referenced in the background, but it's virtually irrelevant because the accumulation of material possessions isn't highly valued or respected. Social status isn't determined by wealth but rather by achievement and merit.

Now you're probably thinking, that's all very good, but I have to pay my bills; I have to eat. And you're right. I've been there. It's a catch-22; you can't forget about money until you have enough money to take care of yourself. But it comes back into focus when you look at this problem from the point of view of your mission.

WHAT DOES MONEY DO FOR YOU?

I'm a massive fan of superheroes. I know they inhabit the realm of fantasy, but I've always believed they present excellent examples for improving one's reality. They represent ideals to which almost all of us aspire, and they are a perfect illustration of what it looks like to devote yourself to a mission.

Now ask yourself: what do superheroes have to do with money? I can't think of many examples of superheroes craving money or devoting themselves to gaining it. Can you imagine Superman using all of his amazing powers simply to get money? Or what about Spider-Man? Maybe Tony Stark is an exception to this in the first *Iron Man* movie, but even he quickly saw how futile and unfulfilling that way of life was. Obsession with money is usually a characteristic of villains, not heroes. For a person with their head screwed on right, money isn't a mission—it's a tool that can sometimes help them achieve their mission.

I saw it during my career in the martial arts, in which I was exposed to a wide variety of people from all walks of life. Very often (but not always), the people I met who had devoted their lives purely to making money and viewed it as an end rather than a means were varying combinations of boring and miserable. Instead of focusing their energies on service, growth, enjoyment, or the use of their gifts, they spent their time chasing something ultimately unfulfilling. After all, when does anyone ever decide they have "enough" money?

Don't get me wrong—money is an important part of the game of life. (The next time somebody tells you money is not important to him, ask him for his wallet.) Be responsible with your money. Spend it wisely and manage it well. But don't become enslaved by it. It's a tool that should serve you, not the other way around. And if you base your sense of self-worth on it, you are almost certainly going to get burned or wake up one day with regrets.

Chasing money for money's sake is very inefficient. And that's because nobody really wants money. They might think they do, but the truth is that what they really want are the things they believe money can buy, like security, power, sex appeal, freedom, or adventure. But I've started to learn that while money can facilitate or enhance some of those things, it's invariably never the creator of them.

And remember that the most valuable things you have in your life were given to you for free. In fact, they are so priceless that trying to put a monetary value on them is almost insulting. I can guarantee that if you're truly intelligent, you wouldn't part with the things that really count for any amount of money.

Don't believe me? How much for your body? What is a lifetime supply of oxygen worth to you? How much would you pay for the love of your parents, or how much would your children need to pay you for yours? What do you think Steve Jobs would have said if someone asked him toward the end of his life if his fortune was worth his health?

HOW WE MAKE MONEY MATTERS

I once asked one of my most successful friends what money meant to him. He told me, "It's just a way of keeping score. It's how I know I'm playing the game well." He wasn't fixated on it. He was focused on giving his all, excelling in his work, and being the very best version of himself. The money came as a result, just as it will for you if you do the same.

Every time I create a product or a service that I feel called to make, I not only have fun doing so, but it results in a financial windfall. In contrast, every time I've entered a project with the sole intention of making money from it, it's had a mediocre reception and not been nearly as profitable as anticipated.

But let me make one thing crystal clear: the "do what you love" mantra has shortcomings, too. I love playing Xbox, but nobody is going to pay me to do that (at this point). There has to be at least a potential pipeline for income associated with the thing you choose to do. And you have to be great at it to have any chance of turning it into something that supports you. So don't think about doing what you love, but about doing what's aligned with your mission, what you have the potential to be great at, and what people are willing to pay for.

The energy from which money is created colors it forever. If you acquire wealth through crooked or deceitful means, it will be tainted with that energy and will likely bring karmic retribution in the form of some negative event, or you'll pay a heavy toll psychologically. I used to be friends with two millionaires who I later found out had built their fortunes through dishonesty. I remember both of them shared the defining trait of being unable to sleep at night.

With the exception of psychopaths and sociopaths, almost everyone instinctively knows this. That's why we have the concepts of "blood money" and "dirty money," and most of us go out of our way to avoid engaging with either. Most of us understand these concepts, but not many of us are familiar with another, similar phenomenon that is nearly as damaging: the effect of money acquired through work that makes you feel inauthentic or unappreciated.

Money that comes to you as a result of these things is unlikely to bring you much joy. I've met many people who were making $250,000 per year working jobs they hated. Many of them were carrying credit card debt because they were wasting so much money trying to spend away the pain. So do everything in your power to make sure the money you earn is good money, happy money. Earn it through activities aligned with your mission and performed with a joyful spirit.

MONEY WILL NOT SOLVE ALL YOUR PROBLEMS

In my late twenties, when I was a struggling jiu jitsu coach living hand to mouth and trying to figure out how to solve the riddle of financial freedom, one of my mentors gave me a very powerful insight.

He said, "You think that when you have money, all of your problems will be gone, but that's delusional. Yes, money solves some problems, but it also brings with it a whole batch of others that you cannot possibly imagine until it happens to you."

I can promise you that if you're unhappy with a little money, you're going to be just as unhappy or even more so when you have a lot. Money, like celebrity and power, is just an amplifier—it amplifies who you already are and magnifies any problems inside yourself that you leave unaddressed.

It pays dividends (pun intended) to build your life around the things that intrinsically bring happiness—things like true connection, service, love, growth, and experience. If your money isn't going toward those things, it's time to rethink your priorities.

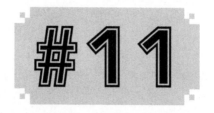

RECONNECT WITH NATURE

——— ★ ★ ★ ———

> *Look deep into nature, and then you will understand everything better."*
>
> **—Albert Einstein**

WE LIVE IN a technological bubble of screens and gadgets. These amazing devices have, in many ways, made our lives far easier and more convenient. But they have also come with a great cost. At the price of unprecedented access to knowledge and opportunity, we also face continual information overload and confusion.

The ability to engage in abstract thought is one of our greatest gifts as humans. It's also a point of weakness. Everything on a screen, regardless of the resolution or subject matter, is just an abstraction.

So when you spend eight hours a day looking at your phone, computer, tablet, or TV, you're spending most of your waking life in a false world. I don't say that with any value judgment imposed; some of these worlds are incredibly entertaining and informative and improve the quality of our lives. But they're not real. No matter how vivid the images and videos appear, they are always going to be pale reflections of reality.

For many, the modern world is characterized by a lack of connection. The countless distractions of our always-on twenty-first-century life have robbed us of the clarity and peace that come from self-knowledge and true connection to nature and others. Scientific materialism—the principle that the tangible, physical world is the only one that exists—has severed the bonds between mind and spirit. We are disconnected from the natural world, including Mother Earth and, in many cases, our own bodies.

Among all the animals, man alone has the unique position that he is both a part of nature and has also transcended it. But nature and our interaction with it are now even more important than they have ever been.

I'm not suggesting you forgo all the comforts and conveniences of modern life. The idea of living off the grid is highly romanticized, and its proponents often downplay or ignore the wondrous human experiences that only modern civilization can facilitate. Anybody who tells you that life was better two hundred years ago has never experienced dysentery, malnutrition, exposure, and other hardships that we can barely fathom today, but that our ancestors lived with on a daily basis.

The intelligent man knows he can have it all—the benefits of both a connection to the natural world and the mastery of technology. He finds the balance between the two.

NATURAL NEEDS

First, the bad news: your comfortable, safe home and high-speed internet connection come with a price. Namely, that spending increasing amounts of time inside or in front of a screen cuts you off from the natural part of yourself.

It's been my experience that if I spend too much time interacting with machines, I start to become almost machine-like in my interactions, and my thought processes become overtly mechanical. Sometimes thinking in this manner is beneficial, but only for brief periods and specific tasks because it comes at the expense of cognitive flexibility and creativity, which are critical to maintaining real-life relationships.

The natural world has been the antidote that's worked for me, and it will work for you, too. Its rawness, unpredictability, and organic beauty are the counterbalance to our man-made world of hard angles and logic. (Did you know, for example, that there are generally no straight lines in nature?)

So what is there in nature that can help cure maladies that stem from spending all day indoors? Well, fresh air is obviously important, but even more important is sunshine. Being under fluorescent lighting is terrible for you. It negatively affects your circadian rhythms, which can lead to poor sleeping patterns and a host of other health issues.

Sunlight is also vital to the creation of another essential nutrient, vitamin D. Your body synthesizes this hugely important substance from sunlight. Except during the summer months, the skin makes little if any vitamin D from the sun at latitudes above thirty-seven degrees north or below thirty-seven degrees south of the equator. People who live in these areas are at relatively greater risk for vitamin D deficiency.

I do not agree with Western medicine's current stance, which has scared us into believing that sunlight is invariably cancerous and detrimental to health, so much so that you need to coat yourself in SPF 100 if you're going to walk by an open window. Yes, the sun is a hugely powerful entity and it should be respected. I wouldn't stand out in the sun in the Arizona desert at midday during the summer without any sort of protection, and if there were a history of melanoma in my family, I'd be extremely careful while spending a lot of time outdoors. But just as with exercise, think of sunlight as something your body requires. If you don't get enough of a specific nutrient, deficiencies arise, which lead to disease. Too much of any specific nutrient creates an imbalance and can also lead to illness. Too much sun can be dangerous, but so is insufficient sun.

If spending time outside in the sunshine is not possible because of the climate where you live, I strongly suggest you consider moving if it's at all possible. I'm not going to sugarcoat it: it's much more difficult to be happy and healthy living in climates with very short summers and very little natural light. We are all affected by this to different degrees—after all, only a few of us get Seasonal Affective Disorder (SAD) in winter—but almost all of us feel happier and more optimistic in sunnier climates.

In fact, I've noticed there's a direct causal effect between my mood and how much time I spend inside. With too much time indoors, I start to become irritable and my mood drops. The effect is compounded when that's combined with large swathes of time in front of the computer: not only do I get even more irritable, but I also find it difficult to look people in the eye, and it requires extra energy to be social.

Now think of the average office job and what it's characterized by: long periods spent inside, staring at a computer and, for far too many people, sitting under fluorescent lighting. It's no wonder so many of us are miserable.

Fortunately, there's a simple and effective solution, one that you've been a master at since you were an infant. It's called walking.

GET UP AND MOVE

Solvitur ambulando is Latin for "It is solved by walking." This expression refers to the phenomenon identified by several great men throughout the ages: the clarifying, restorative power of a simple walk.

When I first moved to the United States, I noticed how much less Americans walked compared to Europeans. In Europe, people will happily walk two miles to the station each morning to catch a train to work. Americans will drive five hundred feet to the store to buy a pack of gum.

After a couple of years living in American society, I realized that I too had begun to walk far less. That's when I began to notice a negative impact on my health and mood, with symptoms similar to what I describe above. To combat this, I committed myself to creating the habit of daily walks and quickly worked my way up to five miles per day. The subsequent improvement in my sense of well-being was marked.

Remember, a complex problem requires a simple solution. And what could be simpler than taking a walk when stuck in a complicated psychological quagmire or when depressed from spending too much time in an artificial environment? Regardless of what's troubling me—be it a business concern, relationship tension, or any sort of anxiety—taking a long walk invariably helps.

Why? Among other health benefits, walking causes your body to engage its parasympathetic nervous system. So if you've been stuck in an office all day with your fight-or-flight response going haywire, a long walk will recenter you and signal to your body that the "danger" has passed and it's time to relax.

We also often forget that walking is a highly efficient, safe form of exercise. It's fantastic for the health of your heart, strengthens your bones, and improves your balance. It provides nearly all the benefits of running, but without the drawback of a detrimental impact on your joints.

Finally, walking is a tremendously effective method for getting out of your head. One of my first courses of action when I find myself caught in a mental loop, or when I'm unable to make a breakthrough on a creative project or business problem, is to go for a walk.

Of course, the benefits of walking compound when you walk or hike outdoors. Hiking is the nexus point of walking and spending time in nature. It's one of the best things you can do to restore presence, healing, and problem-solving. I suggest trying to do a hike at least once a month.

Unless you're in snake-infested terrain or navigating treacherous, uneven surfaces, avoid the tendency to keep your eyes on the ground while walking. Looking down keeps you in your head, limiting those psychological benefits. Instead, look at the horizon and take in the panorama. Take a deep breath. Your mental perspectives will expand as your visual one does.

By now we've covered a whole mess of habits to pick up or drop, which I know can be intimidating. To begin (if you haven't already), I suggest you start by committing to the habit of a daily walk that takes you at least partly into nature, even if it's only for fifteen minutes. If you live in a place without any parks or forests nearby, you should consider doing whatever you can to move to a place with some natural environment available. And yes, you should leave your phone at home, or at the very least, put it in airplane mode.

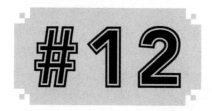

CONSIDER USING PLANT MEDICINE

★ ★ ★

> Many of us who have experienced psychedelics feel very much that they are sacred tools. They open spiritual awareness."
>
> **—Stanislav Grof**

WITHOUT QUESTION, MY dedication and outspoken commitment to plant medicine has always been the most polarizing aspect of my work. It has caused more people to judge me or distance themselves from me than any of my other ostensibly "out there" actions and beliefs. It even (indirectly) led to the end of one of my closest friendships and business relationships.

But despite all that, I still stand by my belief that these substances have extraordinary healing abilities and are massively beneficial for almost everyone when used properly. That's how strongly I feel about this matter.

Your mind might put up a huge amount of resistance against the very thought of this. This is probably due to the thorough job that the misguided War on Drugs has done to brainwash us against the use of psychedelic and hallucinogenic substances. It has done this not only by labeling them illegal, but by categorizing them with other illegal drugs. The result is a totally misleading association between psychedelics and truly dangerous substances like heroin and cocaine.

First, keep in mind that you probably do several drugs every single day of your life, and I'm not referring to pharmaceuticals. A drug is defined as "a medicine or other substance which has a physiological effect when ingested or otherwise introduced into the body." Using that definition, caffeine, nicotine, alcohol, and even many of the foods you eat can be classified as drugs.

And second, it's important to understand that humans have been using natural compounds to change their consciousness for as long as we have existed. It's only very recently that this became a marginalized and criminalized practice.

Yes, certain drugs are very harmful to human health and can, when abused, destroy people's lives and even whole communities. But the mental images most of us have been taught to associate with drug use—junkies with needles in their arms, or losers sniffing coke off toilet seats—are about as far from the reality of plant medicine as anything could possibly be.

The plant medicines I refer to here are not party drugs or life-ruining addictive substances. They are *sacred medicines* that are inextricable from the rituals that accompany them. Their use does not dull the pain of problems but instead forces them to the surface to be processed and dealt with.

These compounds are unmatched in their ability to create radical shifts in perspective, psychological healing, and insight. I've heard it said that one strong Ayahuasca trip is the equivalent to five years of psychotherapy, and I totally believe that—I'm living proof.

THE BENEFITS OF PLANT MEDICINE

My own experience with plant medicine has been deeply healing. It has given me insights into my own psyche, my past, and the nature of reality—things I'm sure I never would have found, let alone deeply understood, from any book, psychologist, or guru.

But don't take it from me. Speak to almost any one of the thousands of individuals who have engaged with plant medicine in a reverent manner and in a controlled setting, and you'll find that almost without exception, they were given direction that guided their mission and knowledge and freed them from past traumas and limiting beliefs.

Perhaps my favorite quote of all time comes from Wayne Dyer: "When you change the way you look at things, the things you look at change." The truth of these words has played out in my life over and over again.

The true power of these substances is their ability to provide fresh perspectives—they help you change the way you look at things. They show you things that it would have been otherwise impossible for your limited ego to see.

Several different plant medicines offer potential for powerful personal development, including peyote, psilocybin, and iboga. I've tried most of them, and the one I feel the most affinity for, and that has allowed for the most breakthroughs and growth, has been ayahuasca. People say a strong ayahuasca trip is like having a telephone conversation with God, and from my experience I can say that's right on point.

The power in ayahuasca and other plant medicines is twofold. First, it provides insights and perspectives into your life, ones that are often so profound and illuminating, they can instantly dissolve negative mental patterns that might have been holding you back for years.

Second, they make you what author Gordon White calls "bulletproof." They give you a glimpse behind the veil and a firsthand experience of the metaphysical realm. This leads to knowledge (not belief!) that there is more to life than just this physical world and, more importantly, more to you than just a physical body. This understanding provides a source of great courage and figurative invincibility.

WORDS OF CAUTION

Keep in mind that these substances are illegal in many places and that their use is not without potential danger. Make sure to do your research properly and choose experienced, qualified guides if you do decide to walk this path.

I've also seen people go too far down the rabbit hole with ayahuasca and plant medicine. This comes from the mistaken belief that any medicine or drug can be the solution to all your problems. Remember, these substances are just tools. They can facilitate your growth and healing, but only if you do the work of self-reflection, introspection, and integration, all of which are necessary both before and after any ceremony or experience.

Don't forget why you started down this path in the first place—in order to finally live fully. So the real power comes from your willingness to change. If you find yourself becoming reliant on these substances, you know you've missed the mark and it's time to pull back and get some space from them.

If you feel a calling to work with plant medicine in a safe environment and supportive setting, check out the retreats that I hold several times per year by following the link at the end of this book.

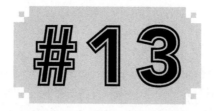

FOLLOW A SLEEP RITUAL

★ ★ ★

> "Sleep is that golden chain that ties health and our bodies together."
>
> **—Thomas Dekker**

I REMEMBER AS a kid that sleep used to be a punishment. Being sent to bed early was one of the worst things that could happen to me. Now I consider it the ultimate reward.

It's my current perspective that quality sleep is the foundation of good health, even more important than nutrition and exercise. Due to the expansion of my business commitments and the constant jet lag from my demanding travel schedule, sleep has become one of the most precious commodities in my life.

The Puritan work ethic, which has done fantastic things for the West and allowed the creation of a great culture, has some drawbacks. One of them is that it associates sleep with laziness and thus causes people to feel guilty for craving and enjoying something that not only makes them healthier and happier, but ultimately more productive too.

In fact, there is a tendency in our society to minimize the importance of sleep and in some cases even vilify it. The "grind" culture exalts the practice of burning the candle at both ends and surviving on as little sleep as possible. Its adherents churn out idiotic slogans like "I'll sleep when I'm dead." With an attitude like that, you'll be dead pretty soon. Or at the very least, you'll feel like you are.

If you choose to live an extraordinary life, you will be placing extraordinary demands on both your physiology and your psyche. The only way that both of these can recuperate and regenerate enough to allow you to continue along this path is if you get consistent, quality sleep.

Think of sleep as the start of your day, not the end of it. It sets the tone for your waking hours. You know the difference in your ability to handle stress, think clearly, and perform efficiently on days following a great night's sleep.

Fortunately, I came to understand this relatively early in life, and as a result I embarked on a lifelong quest to maximize the consistency and quality of my sleep. I have developed what I call "the sleep ritual"—a series of practices and habits that, when implemented, all but guarantees me a great night's sleep. Several of my clients have also used it to great effect. It has several steps and is quite involved, but because of the value I place on my sleep, the effort is well worth it.

THE SLEEP RITUAL

The process begins approximately one hour before bedtime and in the following sequence:

1. **Take a warm shower or bath.**

Warm water has a calming and relaxing effect on both the mind and body and will help to prepare you for sleep.

2. **Turn off all screens.**

Televisions, computers, and mobile phones are all stimulating to the mind, and stimulation and good sleep are not compatible.

3. **Take a sleep-enhancing supplement stack.**

The compounds I have experimented with that seem to be the most effective are, in no particular order:

- ✪ CBD (topical)

- ✪ Magnesium oil

- ✪ Lemon balm

- ✪ Zinc picolinate

- ✪ L-Theanine

- ✪ GABA

Don't take them all at once initially, because then you'll have no idea what is working for you and what isn't. Instead, introduce them one at a time, paying close attention to how they affect you, and try them in combination to discover what works best for your body. Follow the dosage instructions on the supplement.

4. **Stretch for 20 minutes.**

Stretching calms the body by relaxing your muscles and causing your brain to release GABA—a neurotransmitter that decreases activity in your nervous system.

5. **Meditate for 20 minutes.**

Slowing your mind down before bed not only makes it easier to fall asleep, but also makes that sleep deeper and more restfully.

6. **Get in bed and read some fiction for 10–15 minutes.**

Reading fiction will assist your entry into the hypnagogic state, which precedes sleep.

Now, I get that's a lot of stuff to do. I don't do all of the steps myself every night—usually just a couple of them. But if my sleep quality has dropped or I have a big day coming up, I do the whole sequence to guarantee that I wake up refreshed and start my day from a position of strength.

In addition to the sleep ritual, here are some tips that have made a big improvement to my sleep and the sleep of my clients:

Fix Your Environment

A cool, dark room has been clinically proven best for sleep. Turn off or cover all light sources, including the little red LEDs on TVs and other appliances. If you don't yet have blackout blinds in your room, invest in them—they're worth every cent.

Tape Your Mouth

This one is going to sound weird, but every night just before I shut my eyes, I tape my mouth closed using micropore medical tape.

The idea is based on the work of Doctor Konstantin Buteyko, founder of the Buteyko Method. Dr. Buteyko believed breathing through the mouth caused health issues and taping the mouth at night created a system to alleviate respiratory conditions and improve health. What's more, mouth taping completely eliminates snoring, and several people swear it has cured their sleep apnea.

I can say without hesitation that this has been one of the most effective practices I've found, and has led to astounding improvements in both my sleep and overall health.

Avoid Caffeine

Even if you're one of those weird people who can drink a cup of coffee right before you go to sleep, it doesn't mean you should. Caffeine is a stimulant, and even if it doesn't prevent you from going to sleep, it has been shown to shorten total sleep time and deep sleep time, decrease perceived sleep quality, and cause more frequent awakenings.

If you absolutely can't survive without caffeine, try not to consume it after noon. And keep in mind that several nootropic compounds can give you much better effects than coffee does, but without any of the side effects. My own nootropic formula, BDNF, includes several of these compounds.

Wake Naturally

Where you wake up within the sleep cycle is almost as important as how much quality sleep you get. Ideally you want to wake up at the end of a sleep cycle because being jarred awake mid-cycle usually makes you feel like absolute crap.

If at all possible, try to wake up naturally without an alarm clock. This can usually be done if you get enough sleep by going to bed earlier. If this is not an option for you, look into getting an app or smart alarm clock that can wake you gradually and at the correct phase in the sleep cycle.

Take Naps

Do not underestimate the power of napping. We have been trained to believe that daylight is for working only, but for most of our history, humans have existed using polyphasic sleep cycles. In some parts of the world, an afternoon siesta is still a common (albeit dying) practice.

It's been my experience that a twenty-to-sixty-minute nap in the early afternoon increases my productivity, creativity, and sense of well-being. This is backed by plenty of medical research on the subject. Be careful not to nap for too long, though—too much sleep during the day will leave you feeling groggy and compromise your evening rest.

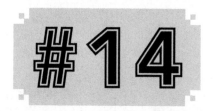

PRIORITIZE & CULTIVATE FOCUS

★ ★ ★

> *I don't care how much power, brilliance or energy you have, if you don't harness it and focus it on a specific target, and hold it there, you're never going to accomplish as much as your ability warrants."*
>
> **—Zig Ziglar**

IF YOU WANT to create something of quality in your life, no matter what it is (e.g., a business, a skill, a relationship), it will require extended periods of focus. There's no getting around it: focusing is a prerequisite for achieving anything of value. Focus and concentration are also prerequisites for being one with the present moment.

The best analogy I've heard that explains the importance of focus is that of sunlight and a magnifying glass. If you place a piece of paper in the sun, it's unlikely to catch fire. But if you use a magnifying glass to focus some of the sun's rays onto a specific point on the paper, very soon it'll be set ablaze.

Think of your energy and time as the sunlight. If they are spent in a diffuse manner and scattered over many tasks, they will be weak and ineffective. But if you use your will to focus, there are few obstacles that you will not be able to "burn through."

The ability to focus has become the most valuable (and scarce) commodity in twenty-first-century life. We live in an age of unlimited distraction, and if you don't have strategies to counter the constant bombardment of "concentration thieves," your output and results will be mediocre at best.

The efficiency found in focus also frees you to work less. Four hours of focused, undistracted work beats twelve hours of watered-down effort snatched between web-surfing and texting any day of the week.

There are several keys to an increased ability to focus. Here are the ones that have helped me and my clients the most.

1. DECLUTTER YOUR ENVIRONMENT

We all have far too much stuff. The unspoken mantra of the last several generations has been "acquire, acquire, acquire." Generally, buying new stuff brings a very brief, very shallow rush of enjoyment and novelty. This is quickly replaced by apathy toward the item, which very often leads to it being shelved in a cupboard or stored away in a garage somewhere.

Deep down, we know we don't need a lot of the stuff surrounding us, but we hold onto it because of misplaced nostalgia or fear we'll need it later, not because we enjoy these things or get use out of every last item. And your environment (home, office, etc.) is a pretty accurate reflection of your mind. If it's cluttered with too many things and lots of unused stuff, your mind is the same—overloaded with too many thoughts and stale ideas.

One of the roles of the active male principle in the world is to impose order on chaos. That's why man creates civilization—he is imposing order on the chaos he finds in nature. That's why tidying your environment and creating functional spaces feels so fulfilling: it's literally one of your "prime directives" as a man.

When the spaces in your life are clean and uncluttered, the energy flows. You become more creative, more relaxed, and more efficient. I've truly taken this to heart, and it has worked wonders in my life. My home and office are all kept exceptionally neat—there is nothing wasted or out of place. My years as a digital nomad, spent traveling the world with all I owned in a backpack and a duffel bag, proved to me that you do not need much to be extremely happy. With the exception of a few pieces of art, everything has a definite purpose and is used frequently. As a result, these are places that are conducive to both relaxation and quality work.

Keep in mind that decluttering is a continual process. Every couple of months, I do a mini-spring cleaning, giving or throwing away anything that isn't being used or that I instinctively feel no longer serves me. Unsurprisingly, I notice upticks in my output and mental well-being immediately after clearing out my space. Think of it like hitting "refresh" on the environment around you. As we all know, it's beneficial to restart our devices, so why should it be any different for the space and the things around you?

Don't confuse elimination of clutter with extreme minimalism. I like nice things and own several fine objects myself, but I am extremely conscious of the pitfalls of accumulating more than I need to live a balanced life. For example, when something new enters my home, it usually means something old has to go. It's far better to own a few quality belongings that you treasure and use than a hoard of low-quality crap that sits gathering dust.

I believe there's a lot of truth in the line from the film *Fight Club*: "Sooner or later the things you own start to own you." Indeed, it's been shown that people who spend their money on experiences rather than things are far happier than those who do the opposite. So the next time you're tempted to purchase a consumer good, ask yourself if you *really* need it. If the answer is no, consider instead spending the money on an experience that you've wanted to have for a while—you'll be glad you did.

2. ELIMINATE DISTRACTIONS

It's not just about eliminating extraneous stuff. Even more important is eliminating distractions. It was only when I began to be ruthless about the distractions in my life that things really began to take off for me, particularly when it came to business.

Your phone and computer are tools. Make sure you are the one using them, and that you are not being used *by* them. I suggest you turn off all but the most essential notifications on them. As Cal Newport described in his fantastic book *Digital Minimalism*, each time your focus is stolen by one of these notifications, it takes time and energy to get it back, greatly reducing your efficiency.

But remember, you're trying to be your best self, not just your most efficient self. When you're spending time in the company of another person, commit to not using your phone in their presence. Honor the person there in front of you by giving them your full attention and focus. You'll differentiate yourself from 99 percent of humanity, you'll get more out of the encounter, and they'll feel flattered and appreciated.

3. DO ONE THING AT A TIME

There is no such thing as multitasking. It literally doesn't exist except within the world of computing. Train yourself into the habit of giving your full attention to whatever task you are doing, no matter how menial. If you're speaking to a friend on the phone, don't surf the web at the same time. If you're writing an email, don't try to watch a TV show in the background. The effects of focusing on what you're doing include increased attention span, more efficient use of time, and more enjoyment of each activity you spend your time on.

4. EMBRACE ROUTINE

Don't confuse routine for monotony. By reducing the number of low-level choices you need to make, routines free up your brain's processing power to be used for more important decisions and thoughts.

Here's an example of this phenomenon that I learned from my friend Johnny FD, the founder of digital nomad culture. Each evening, I lay out my clothes for the next day, then spend a few minutes reviewing and planning the tasks I want to complete on waking. When I wake up the following morning, no time or energy is wasted contemplating what I'm going to wear or what needs to get done.

Routines and habits have a lot of overlap. I cover morning routines in greater detail in chapter 19.

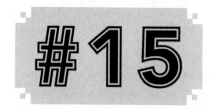

OPTIMIZE YOUR TESTOSTERONE

★ ★ ★

> *Testosterone to me is so important for a sense of well-being when you get older."*
>
> **—Sylvester Stallone**

IN MY LATE thirties, I noticed a pretty drastic change in myself, one characterized by both physical and mental syndromes.

Working out, once one of my most beloved pastimes, had become a huge chore and invariably left me chronically stiff and sore the following day. My muscles didn't respond to training the same way they used to, and my metabolism had slowed massively. I also began to lack motivation, and my friends noticed I had become uncharacteristically (and unreasonably) moody.

As somebody who had generally always been happy, ambitious, driven, and strong, this situation was completely unacceptable to me.

I believe that I'm responsible for my own health, so I embarked on an exhaustive search to figure out the cause of these issues. This included a lot of research, visits to doctors, and several supplement regimens. At one point I was even convinced I had a thyroid issue and tried thyroid medication, which helped a little, but only briefly.

Finally, through a specific blood test, I was finally able to pinpoint the cause of the issue: low testosterone.

My doctor prescribed testosterone replacement therapy (TRT), which consisted of two shots of testosterone (Cypionate) per week. Initially, I was reluctant to start the course of medication. I didn't like the thought of being dependent on something for the rest of my life, nor the idea of not being "natural." But most of all, I just didn't want to admit to myself that I was not the man I used to be.

I got over these reservations after doing extensive research, and eventually I came to accept this one key understanding: life was horrible with low testosterone, and it had to change. The relatively low risks and blow to my ego from feeling dependent on medication were well worth the potential upsides of renewed health and vigor.

Two weeks after starting replacement therapy, I felt better than I had in years. I started to actively look forward to working out, particularly lifting weights. My outlook on life improved dramatically, as did my sex drive (I subsequently found out that until the advent of SSRIs, testosterone used to be prescribed for depression). What's more, I started to become firmer with my boundaries, and as a result, several toxic relationships in my life began to dissolve.

In short, TRT has been a miracle in my life and one of the best decisions I've ever made.

GLOBAL EPIDEMIC

If your testosterone is low, it's important to understand that it's nothing to be ashamed of and you definitely aren't alone. For reasons beyond the understanding of science and medicine, men's testosterone levels have been declining by 1 percent per year since the 1970s. This means a forty-year-old man today has a testosterone level of only half that of his father's when he was the same age.

Some attribute this decline to increasingly sedentary lifestyles; others claim it's caused by pollution and the xenoestrogenic effect of all the plastics in our environment. The cause could be a combination of all of these, or it could be none of them. The truth is that nobody knows why it's happening, just that it is, and at epidemic levels.

THE IMPORTANCE OF TESTOSTERONE

The truth is, if your testosterone has been low for some time, you probably don't even remember what it was like to truly feel well. Here's a list of just some of the benefits of having healthy testosterone levels:

- ✪ Reduced inflammation

- ✪ Increased muscle mass

- ✪ Improved cognition

- ✪ Increased libido

✪ Stronger bones

✪ Elevated/stabilized mood

In short, almost every positive aspect of being a man is either totally dependent on or greatly modulated by testosterone.

NATURAL ALTERNATIVES

Before engaging in a medical intervention, I believe it's usually best to address health issues with lifestyle changes and natural alternatives. In the case of low testosterone, there are certain things you can do to address the issue, several of which are covered in this book. These include:

✪ Getting adequate sunlight

✪ Optimizing your sleep

✪ Engaging in frequent resistance training

✪ Eliminating alcohol

✪ Avoiding pornography

✪ Supplementing your diet with vitamin D3

If you believe your levels are low, I suggest the following approach:

1. Get your bloodwork done so you can get an accurate metric of what's going on. Make sure the lab tests both "free" and "total" testosterone.

2. If your levels are below the normal range, start by cleaning up your lifestyle for three months, following the advice in this book.

3. After three months, get your levels checked again. If there is no significant improvement, make an appointment with an endocrinologist or medical professional who has experience with TRT.

If you have a hunch that your testosterone might be low and you would like to read a detailed and comprehensive resource on how to tackle the issue, I recommend *The Testosterone Optimization Therapy Bible* by my friend, Jay Campbell. It covers pretty much everything you need to know and will allow you to make an educated decision without being at the mercy of a doctor who may not be familiar with TRT and its benefits.

Today I'm happier, healthier, and stronger than I've ever been, and that's in large part due to the miracle of TRT. Don't miss out on this life-changing medicine because of your ego or fear of others' opinions.

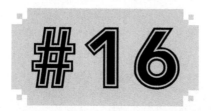

BECOME COURAGEOUS

★ ★ ★

66 *Everything you want is on the other side of fear."*
—George Addair

THIS SHOULD BE obvious, but there's more to a man than a healthy body and a successful lifestyle. So if you truly want to reach your full potential, you'll need to look inward as well. Among other things, a man needs to be brave, reflective, and resilient, and these next chapters contain some wisdom I've accumulated along my journey to help you cultivate these important qualities.

My favorite quote from Terrence McKenna, one of the greatest minds of the twentieth century, is "Nature loves courage." Nature loves courage because it is *the* prerequisite for growth. And growth is the prime directive of all life.

This is a strange quirk built into the nature of the human experience: you cannot go to the next level in any area of your life without overcoming some fear. There is no exception to this. This fear exists because any decision that could lead to growth has the potential for undesirable consequences. And because nobody can make your decisions for you, the responsibility for these consequences rests on your shoulders alone.

Every major breakthrough in my life has come after making (and acting on) a decision that caused at least some level of anxiety. And to give myself that chance to grow, I had to get over my need to feel secure.

FORGET SECURITY

> *Life is either a daring adventure or nothing. Security does not exist in nature, nor do the children of men as a whole experience it. Avoiding danger is no safer in the long run than exposure."*
> **—Hellen Keller**

Security is an illusion. Nothing is guaranteed in life. As I write this, millions of people who held onto shitty jobs at the expense of their happiness and self-actualization because they provided "security" are unemployed in the wake of the COVID-19 pandemic.

Stop using security as the primary factor on which you base your decisions. You've come from a long line of adventurous and brave humans who conquered a harsh, unforgiving planet and overcame war, famine, and a million other challenges.

They didn't do this so you could be "secure" in your climate-controlled townhouse, drinking cinnamon lattes while watching others take risks on television. They did it so you could reach even further and do great things—things that are characterized by uncertainty and demand courage.

Take calculated risks. Reach for what you want out of life.

THE COURAGE FORMULA

We all have different amounts of natural courage. Some are just naturally braver than others. But regardless of where you are now, you can increase your current level of courage. Think of it as a skill like any other—all you need is dedication and practice.

Three key understandings will assist you in the development of this skill. I call the application of these understandings the Courage Formula:

1. **You must go to where the fear is.**

This means exactly what you think it does. You have to train yourself to actively seek out circumstances and activities that you're afraid of and engage with them. Not only will this help you to overcome those fears, but it will likely also lead you to some of the most rewarding experiences of your life.

2. **Courage is a reward.**

Let's pretend there's a fear scale that starts at 0 (no fear at all) and goes up to 100 (absolute, abject terror). By facing any activity on that scale head-on, you will be rewarded with the equivalent amount of courage.

For example, let's say skydiving is at a 60 on the fear scale for you. By facing it and jumping out of that plane, you will gain 60 units of courage in your "emotional bank account."

Sure, it's an arbitrary scale, and the numbers you assign don't have any basis in reality, but the act of assigning the numbers adds an element of gamification to something that is otherwise overly serious and foreboding. And although they may be intangible, the rewards of courage are definitely real.

3. **Starting small is key.**

It's important to understand that courage is like a muscle in that it becomes stronger with use. And just as with any muscle, it's not the best idea to start lifting the heaviest weights right away—you should progressively work up to them.

So start by facing small fears and work your way up—stuff that is 5–10 on the scale, even if it's something as trivial as asking out the cute barista who works at your local coffee shop. Through this progressive exposure therapy, it will eventually become possible to face even the biggest fears that have been holding you back your whole life.

CONQUERING THE GREATEST OF ALL FEARS

There are two strong fears that you must overcome to become fully self-actualized. The first of these is often called the "root of all fears" because if you dig down into any anxiety deeply enough, you'll find this sitting at the heart of it—the fear of death.

The fear of death is powerful because it's tied to the ego's fear of dissolution and of things it cannot totally prepare for or control.

The only way to overcome this great fear is to meditate on your death and fully accept it. Literally set some time aside to stop and think about it without distraction. Say to yourself, I am going to die one day, and really think about what that means.

One day you will cease to be, at least in your current form. And nobody knows what will happen to your consciousness at that point. It might disappear entirely, it might be reincarnated in another form, or it might transition to a different realm. Nobody knows, and anyone who tells you otherwise is lying to you. Acknowledge and embrace this paradox of certainty and uncertainty. It is absolutely certain you will die, and it is absolutely uncertain what will happen at that point. These are two of the few indisputable truths that anybody can offer you.

Once you internalize these and make peace with them, the fear of death loses a lot of power over you. It is pointless being afraid of something you have no control over. A much more real and valid fear is of having lived a life of unrealized potential. If you are going to be motivated by fear, that's a much healthier one.

The second "master" fear is perfectly described in the following quote by the spiritual teacher Osho:

> *The greatest fear in the world is the opinion of others, and the moment you are unafraid of the crowd, you are no longer a sheep, you become a lion. A great roar arises in your heart, the roar of freedom."*

The wisdom contained within the above declaration is some of the most powerful stuff you will ever encounter.

We are social creatures descended from ancestors who, for millennia, existed within small tribes consisting of 150 people or less. Everybody knew everybody, and if you pissed off or alienated enough people in the tribe, you were expelled into the literal wilderness, which almost always meant certain death. Because of this origin, we are genetically hardwired to be concerned with what the tribe thinks of us. Add constant societal reinforcement from a young age, and it's no surprise that we are predisposed to following the crowd.

But we don't live in that world anymore. Technology and modern society have freed us from reliance on the tribe. You can do just fine on your own, and if your own tribe rejects you, it's never been easier to find another that's more aligned with who you are and what you stand for.

Overcoming this master fear has been a huge challenge in my life and one that I am constantly vigilant about conquering. It's not easy to overcome this, but the rewards for those who do are great. There is a mindset that can loosen the crowd's hold over you, and all it takes is accepting two basic assertions:

1. **Not everybody is supposed to like you.**

Most of us want to be liked by everyone, so we adapt our behavior and our opinions in an attempt to appease our friends and family. The root of this is usually a lack of unconditional love during childhood; most of our parents (often unwittingly) put prerequisites on our behavior for their approval. This people-pleasing, conformist behavior usually results in a life of mediocrity. Just accept this fact for what it is.

Just accept that if you want to have an extraordinary life, you're going to need to do extraordinary things, and this means some people aren't going to like or agree with you.

Another way I've heard this put is if you put yourself or your creations out there, a third of the people are going to love you, a third are going to hate you, and a third aren't going to care either way.

2. **Nobody gives a fuck.**

This is closely related to the above and just as important. I hate to break it to you, but in the lives of pretty much everybody else, you just aren't that important. You take up very little time and space in others' thoughts.

An even harsher truth is that this is even true (to some extent) in the case of the people you love. In reality, you take up far, far less space in the minds of your friends, family, and social circle than you think you do. They devote very little mental energy to you and your life because they're busy thinking of their own problems, dreams, and desires.

THE OPINIONS OF OTHERS

Here's another powerful quote:

> *I used to worry about the opinions of others until I tried to pay my bills with them."*

All those people whose opinions you are so concerned with — are they going to be sitting next to you, consoling you when you're an old man on your deathbed, regretting all the things you didn't do for fear of being judged?

Think of how many decisions you've made in your life based on the thoughts or opinions of others. If you're honest with yourself, you'll realize it's been the vast majority of them. It's time for that to change. If you want to live a life of greatness, you'll have to make your own opinion the most important one in your life. This is *your* life.

Remember, you probably don't want those who judge you in your life anyway. True friendship and love is accepting who you are. As long as your viewpoints or actions aren't harmful to others, what gives anybody else the right to pass judgment on them?

I remember before I got my first tattoo, several people told me it would cause people to make assumptions about me and limit my job choices. My first thought at the time was, if somebody judges me for having a tattoo on my arm, then the tattoo has done me a great service by actively filtering that person out of my life. And I still believe I hit the nail on the head with that assessment.

One of the guiding principles of my life is a concept I formulated that I call the Law of 180. The Law of 180 states: "To attain the peaks of the human experience, look at what the crowd is doing, and do the exact opposite." That is, turn 180 degrees from the direction everyone else is going.

Every one of the truly successful, happy, and actualized people I know hit the same pivotal moment at least once: the part of their story at which people were telling them they were wrong. To achieve anything noteworthy, you too will have to come to a point where your course of action seems at odds with the tribe, or at least with the vast majority of society.

Want to be fit and healthy? Don't sit on the stationary bike reading the newspaper or eat three meals per day. Lift weights and do intermittent fasting instead.

Want to be wealthy? Don't work at a job for forty years and count on your 401(k). Start a business instead.

Want to have a calm, clear mind? Instead of watching four hours of TV every day, meditate, do yoga, and spend time in nature.

Want to profit from the stock market? Buy when everybody else is selling.

The list goes on and on. Watch the crowd — see where their attention (or hysteria) is directed. Now look 180 degrees in the opposite direction. The knowledge, solution, or fulfillment you seek is that way.

And don't stop at the actions of the crowd. Question *all* existing structures. Just because something has been done a certain way for a long time does not necessarily make it right, beneficial, or efficient. Instead of fearing what other people will think, use their thoughts as an inspiration for what *not* to do.

GO BEYOND THOUGHT

Don't think—feel."

—Bruce Lee

Rationale and logic are some of mankind's greatest gifts and have had an enormous, generally positive impact on civilization. But for the individual, they can only take us so far.

Taking courageous action may not always make sense from a rational perspective. Courage is a phenomenon that has more to do with the realm of feeling than thought. Your mind wants to maintain the status quo. It doesn't want you to grow because growth requires change, and change is risky.

This is one of the many ways in which women are often far superior to men. They generally have much more refined and heightened awareness of their instincts and internal states. There's a reason women's intuition is so valued by truly successful men.

Learn to trust the inner voice that speaks from the heart, not the head. Taking the high-paying job might be the logical, safe choice, but if on a deep level you just *know* it's not what you want, it doesn't *feel* right, then it will almost certainly result in a less-than-stellar outcome.

Learning to truly feel your emotions and cultivating the courage to trust your inner voice are two of the most powerful and rewarding things you will ever do. For further information on this topic, read *You Can Have it All* by Arnold Patent and *Letting Go: The Pathway to Surrender* by David R. Hawkins.

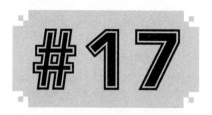

#17

SEE THE MIRROR

★ ★ ★

> *Life is an echo. What you send out comes back. What you sow, you reap. What you give, you get. What you see in others exists in you."*
>
> **—Zig Ziglar**

CONTINUING OUR JOURNEY inward, let's talk a bit about just who and what it is you're working to improve.

The more I study life, the more I believe the theory that we are living in some sort of simulation. I cannot say with any degree of certainty who or what created this simulation or why it exists, although I do have several theories that I won't go into here. But if we are indeed in a simulation, that changes everything we know about . . . well, everything.

The human experience is nothing more than an incredibly sophisticated game that is played out within this simulation. Simulations all have certain characteristics and a set of parameters, and games all have rules. While I believe life is inherently a mystery and its ultimate meaning is unknowable,

I also believe that many of these parameters and rules can be discovered, and that it is indeed wise to learn and understand them so you can become the best possible player of the game.

The most powerful insight I've discovered through my own experience and relentless observation of life is that the simulation we exist in, when taken in the context of the human experience, has the characteristics of a mirror—it is constantly reflecting who and what we are back at us. This is evident everywhere, but especially when it comes to the Law of Attraction.

Now, the Law of Attraction is a poorly understood, often misused principle. That's because the vast majority of people don't know the truth behind it, which is that you attract what you *are*, not what you *want*.

REFLECTIONS

Here's an example of that misconception: Billy reads *The Secret* and is inspired by the Law of Attraction. He likes the idea that he can easily get what he wants with minimal effort except for a few specifically directed thoughts. He spends several months sitting on his couch, thinking about a million dollars, expecting to attract it to himself. When the riches don't magically appear, he gives up in frustration.

What's Billy doing wrong? He does not understand how the Mirror really works, and thus his application of the Law of Attraction is flawed.

The first thing to understand is that the Universe will only ever meet you halfway. When you take action, Creation will rise up to support you, but it will not do everything for you. Secondly, if we look closely at Billy and *who he is*, we will see that he is more likely than not embodying neediness, desire, and lack. Therefore, that is what the simulation will reflect back to him.

If he instead studied the habits of the wealthy and started to adopt the identity of someone who had earned a million dollars—say, managing his money wisely, being generous, creating value in the world through quality goods and services, etc.—he would start to *feel* wealthy, and the Universe would reflect that back at him through increased opportunities and an increased flow of money into his life.

Here's another example to illustrate the concept of the Mirror. Paul is the guy who is perpetually angry at life, who thinks everyone and everything is out to get him. Because he embodies anger—he literally *is* anger, in a very real sense—the world consistently reflects that back at him and he continually encounters people, circumstances, and events that exacerbate and are conducive to his anger.

This is something of which I am totally convinced at this point. It has gone beyond belief and become knowledge. I don't need theories or philosophies to confirm or deny it—I have experienced the truth of it far too many times to require either of those.

Here's an example from my own life: several years ago I got into the bad habit of downloading films and music illegally. I never felt great about it but always managed to rationalize it away, using one excuse or another. At the time, I was also selling my own digital jiu jitsu books and videos online. In a moment of clarity, the following thought occurred to me:

How can I expect people to value the things I create if I don't value the ones they create?

At that point I deleted everything in my digital library that I hadn't paid for and made a commitment not to devalue the output of others by consuming it without paying for it. Without anything else changing, almost immediately I noticed an increase in the sales of my own products.

Here's another expression that hints at the truth of the simulation mirror theory: "That which you declare war on, you energize." I saw this demonstrated over and over during my martial arts journey. In fact, one of the earliest lessons I remember receiving from my judo coach when I was seven years old was, "If you push someone, the first thing he will do is push back. And if you pull him, he will pull back against you."

The way you approach life is how it will reflect back at you. What you expect to see will be shown to you. If a person wakes up and goes out into the world believing that life is difficult, short, and ugly and that everybody is out to get him, then that's exactly what his experience will be.

Yet another way I've heard this put is "Whatever you need more of, the solution is to give more of it." If you're lonely and feel you're lacking friends, be friendly to others as much as possible. If you desire love, give love to others. If you want to increase the flow of money into your life, give more money to others.

Once you understand this, you will quickly realize that if you want to have the highest-quality human experience, it only makes sense to embody positive virtues and traits. Of these, I've found that the most powerful is gratitude.

LOOK FOR GRATITUDE

One of the most profound ideas I've ever encountered came from one of the Vedic scriptures. It is the understanding that for a soul, the experience of a human life is very difficult to obtain, and it requires the journey of thousands of incarnations before it is granted. I don't know if that's true, but it always makes me feel profoundly inspired and motivated when I think about it, and it makes me treasure my life even more.

When you reframe your life as the ultimate gift and you are grateful for it and everything in it, including your challenges, you are in essence appreciating the Universe for the great privilege it has granted you. And that gratitude profoundly affects the life that will reflect back to you in the mirror.

What would happen if you gave someone a gift and they complained about it? I'd wager that it's highly unlikely you'd give them another one. But what if they expressed great appreciation for it and thanked you sincerely and profusely?

It's the same with your life. If you see it as a miracle and are grateful for it, and you express that to the Universe, God, or Creation, then he, she, or it is far more likely to shower you with even more blessings.

Most people dwell on what they don't have, which shifts them toward the polarity of scarcity and lack. When they embody this energy, it's not surprising that they continue to perpetuate situations defined by scarcity and lack.

The solution is gratitude, thankfulness for all of the positive things in your life. And there is so, so much to be grateful for, regardless of how grim your current circumstances may seem.

One of the things I get all of my clients to do is spend ten minutes each evening before bed listing five things they are grateful for from the day's events. Most of them start out enjoying the exercise but quickly become frustrated after a few weeks because they run out of things to be grateful for. My answer to them is always, "You're not trying hard enough. There are always more things to be grateful for."

Here are a few that come to my mind with very little effort:

- ✪ The sun and the consistent shower of energy it gives us to support life on this planet.

- ✪ The privilege of being blessed with running water, proper nutrition, and countless entertainment options (unlike most human beings throughout history)

- ✪ My five senses and how incredibly they work to allow me to navigate reality

- ✪ The friends and family in my life who love and support me

- ✪ The skills I've amassed over the course of my life and my ability to use them to make the world a better place

- ✪ The limitless amount of information freely available at my fingertips through the internet

- ✪ The fact that statistically, I live in the safest, most prosperous time in the history of the world

✪ The indescribable sophistication and beauty of the natural world that exists all around me to enjoy

Like any other habit, training yourself to embody and project gratitude will take some time, discipline, and effort on your part. But once it is ingrained in you, it becomes your default as you move through the world, and then life becomes truly magical.

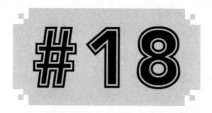

LEARN TO LET GO

★ ★ ★

> *Time doesn't heal emotional pain, you need to learn how to let go."*
>
> **—Roy T. Bennet**

I STAND BY everything I've shared with you in this book as being truthful and accurate from my current perspective. But there are truths, and then there are Truths with a capital T. Unlike ordinary truths, which may shift based on updated information or the introduction of new viewpoints, Truths are timeless, deep "knowings" that, due to a combination of instinct and experience, have transcended the label of "belief."

In all my years of searching, I've found only a small handful of Truths. The Mirror from the previous chapter is one, and what follows is another.

Several years ago I read David R. Hawkins' life-changing book *Letting Go: The Pathway to Surrender*. It had a far-reaching, positive influence on my life and drastically altered the way I move through the world. I found what was shared within to be so profound that the minute I finished it, I returned to the first page and began reading it again. I'm now on my fourth read-through. It's the book I most often give away or recommend to friends and clients, and has been for years now.

In it, Dr. Hawkins explains that the only healthy way to process negative emotions is to feel them in their entirety and then actively let go of them.

Because negative emotions can be so painful and uncomfortable to deal with, and because we've never been informed of this fact or taught how to use it, most of us adopt ineffective and damaging strategies to deal with them instead. We suppress these feelings through distractions, addictions, or acting out in damaging ways.

But emotions are a form of energy, and if that energy is not allowed to flow and ultimately dissipate, it will remain trapped within the psyche, physiology, and spirit of the person who has repressed it. Because like attracts like (and because the world is a mirror), that trapped energy will then cause people, circumstances, and events of a similar energy to appear in the person's life.

Holding onto resentment and other negative emotions is, in my perspective, one of the most self-destructive things a man can do. It's like holding onto a burning coal—the only one who gets burned is you.

If you don't deal with your internal shit, it will keep playing out over and over in your life. Even worse, you'll be powerless to fix it by altering your actions or changing your external circumstances, regardless of how hard you try .

I've seen the truth of this verified countless times in my own experience. Here's an example:

My parents had a terrible, highly dysfunctional marriage. My mother, being emotionally stunted and lacking a healthy way to deal with her own negative feelings regarding the lack of support from my father, would turn to me and vent all of her fear, anger, and frustration. I was just a young child and not equipped to rationally process these painful feelings, so I internalized and ultimately suppressed them. As I became an adult, I compounded the problem by becoming angry and resentful toward both of my parents for allowing this to happen.

For years my romantic relationships were characterized by the same type of conflict that had been the norm in my childhood home. The unaddressed emotions within me were playing out in my circumstances by unconsciously dictating my actions and choices and by causing me to be attracted to people with similar unsolved emotional issues.

It wasn't until I became aware of this and made an active effort to relive those childhood traumas—to feel them in their entirety and then ultimately let go of the anger and resentment associated with them—that the pattern changed.

LET GO OF EXPECTATIONS

In addition to recreating the negativity you've already experienced, holding onto things also prevents you from moving forward in your life and blocks new experiences from flowing toward you. I always imagine this as being similar to Tarzan swinging through the jungle from vine to vine. As he swings forward and grabs the vine in front of him, it cannot pull him forward until he has let go of the vine behind him. If he keeps holding onto it, his momentum will stop entirely.

I've seen this effect many times with my clients. They deeply desire to create a new experience for themselves, whether it be a career change or a body transformation. But because they have been unable to let go of the security of the existing job or set of comfortable habits due to fear of the unknown, they block the entry of new, better things into their lives. Letting go creates space within you—space for new things to enter.

This is especially prevalent when it comes to relationships. People hang onto relationships that no longer serve them because they're afraid of being alone and are thus unable to allow the opportunity for better-suited partners to enter their lives.

Keep in mind that letting go always requires a leap of faith (which takes courage!). There's no way around this. If you hedge your bets, then you aren't truly letting go. Comedian Steve Harvey uses the analogy of skydiving to refer to this phenomenon. In order to be able to have that amazing experience, you have to literally let go of the plane and trust that the parachute will open.

When you are reaching for the next thing, you need to fully accept that what you are letting go of is gone forever. You can't have any remaining attachment to it. God, the Universe, or the market responds only to total commitment—not to hesitant half-steps.

LET GO OF JUDGMENT

Closely related to this is the counterproductive habit of holding onto judgments. A person's judgment of his circumstances is like an energetic glue that holds those circumstances in place. When you let go of the judgments, the circumstances almost always change or dissolve.

Oprah Winfrey perfectly illustrated this in a story she related. In the 1980s, Oprah auditioned for a role in Steven Spielberg's *The Color Purple*. Due to the subject matter of the film, Oprah was very emotionally attached to the idea of being involved in the project. At the time she had no acting experience and was up against several well-known performers for the role. Convinced she had no chance, Oprah got to the point where she just surrendered all of her judgments about the situation and the other actresses. Minutes later, Steven Spielberg called to offer her the role.

Here's another example from my own life: at age thirty-two, I let go of literally everything I had: a lovely home, a decent job, a fantastic social circle, and a girlfriend who adored me. Even though I had it pretty good, I also knew deep down that it could be better. There was a calling within me to expand and explore. I gave up everything—and I mean everything—and purchased a ticket to Thailand with no real plan. Taking that risk and making the space within my life for something fresh and new paid off. The next four years were absolutely incredible, brought with them so many wonderful new experiences and relationships, and ultimately blessed me with everything I had given up and more.

Now admittedly the example above is quite extreme, and you might not be able to take such drastic action right away. But at the very least, you can start with getting rid of some of your stuff.

LET GO OF THINGS

As I mentioned in chapter 14, chances are you own way, way too many things. The recent movement toward minimalism over the last several years has introduced many people to the power of letting go.

We usually hold onto physical things because of a scarcity mindset. When you understand that there's enough for everyone, you are far more likely to give up things you don't need anymore. All that stuff takes up space not only in your environment, but also in your mind.

I'm not a huge fan of reality TV shows, but every so often one of them offers something truly insightful. Marie Kondo, a Japanese lifestyle consultant, shared a phenomenal piece of wisdom on her series *Tidying Up* that has helped me navigate what to keep and what to let go of. When evaluating whether to hold onto something, use only one yardstick: does it spark joy?

When you combine that question with the three-month rule, it's very easy to quickly separate what you truly need to be happy and what's become a drag on your mind and spirit. (The three-month rule states that, with the exception of suitcases, seasonal clothing, and a few other very specific items, if you haven't used something in three months, chances are you can do without it permanently and you should consider parting with it.)

Once you've made it a habit to let go of physical things that no longer serve you, move on to thoughts and then people. You'll be amazed at how much energy you free up in your life and the beautiful new things you allow to flow into it.

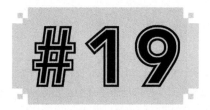

CREATE A POWERFUL ROUTINE

★ ★ ★

> " *Every morning start a new page in your story.* "
> —**Doe Zantamata**

MANKIND'S CREATIONS ARE characterized by a tendency toward entropy. Left alone, they tend to break down and fragment. Consider the example of a house that's left unoccupied for several years: with no outside intervention, it very quickly begins to break down and fall into disarray.

And the same is true for the life of a man: it must constantly be maintained and tended to stay healthy and continue to grow. Your finances, your body, your business, and your relationships will not just take care of themselves. If left alone, they will revert to a state of chaos and eventually break down.

Remember, one of man's greatest gifts is his ability to impose order on the world, and one of the most powerful ways you can use this gift is to create and adhere to routines that serve you in your life. Of these, none is more effective or more conducive to health, wealth, and happiness than a well-planned morning routine.

POWER IN THE MORNING

If you're like I used to be, you probably start your day reaching for your phone and checking your messages, your favorite websites, and the news. You then stumble into the bathroom, get yourself presentable, eat breakfast, and head out toward your place of work.

While this might be an adequate way for the average man to start his engagement with the world, it falls far short of what is required for excellence. (As a side note, if you haven't figured out by now that the news is generally toxic, sensationalist bullshit that generally has no bearing on your existence and that you're better off without it, you really need to do so quickly.)

Those close to me understand that my mornings are sacred to me. I now know that the way my morning goes largely dictates the way my day goes. And the way my days go cumulatively determines the way my life goes. There is absolutely no doubt about it: the days on which I do my upgraded, purposeful morning routine flow more easily and are vastly more enjoyable and productive than the days on which I neglect to do it.

This is my current morning routine, and it has served me very well.

1. **Do 15 minutes of mobility work and light stretching.**

I suggest you start with fifteen to twenty minutes of mobility work and stretching each morning. This connects you to your body and causes positive changes in your brain, which facilitate enhanced learning and performance for the rest of the day.

2. Do 30–45 minutes of meditation.

There's a Buddhist saying that goes "You should meditate for thirty minutes each day, unless you are too busy—then you should meditate for an hour." Starting the day with meditation centers and prepares you for what lies ahead.

3. Do 15 minutes of state priming.

My own coach impressed upon me the importance of this particular practice. State priming is a set of actions that motivate and uplift me, getting me to a place where I know that I'll be taking good energy with me when I go out into the world. It includes listening to inspiring music, reading, and saying affirmations. Most importantly, it includes envisioning my desired future and feeling the emotions associated with the achievement of it.

4. Spend 30 minutes studying Japanese.

At the time of writing this, I'm going through a Japan obsession, so this particular habit is well suited to me, but obviously it doesn't have to be Japanese language study for everyone. Choosing to spend some time in the morning on the acquisition of any skill fosters feelings of empowerment and confidence that will permeate all your other activities during the day.

By now you're probably thinking, what?! Over an hour devoted to a morning routine? That means I'll have to wake up at 5:00 a.m.! I can't do that—I need my sleep. I don't have time for that!

That's a classic excuse, and one that holds absolutely no water whatsoever. You have more than enough time. It's your priorities that need to change. All you need to do is go to bed earlier. Now that might mean you have to miss out on some television, some video games, or an evening at the bar and prioritize your growth and development over entertainment. Are you prepared to do that? Or do you want to be like the other 99.9 percent and fold at the first sign of resistance?

The importance of this routine really can't be overstated. Even if you're a shift worker who has a job that makes this impossible, it's time to start looking for a new job or line of work. The detrimental effects of night shifts on your health are incontrovertible and vastly outweigh any economic benefit they might be providing.

For a deeper dive into the powerful practice of creating a morning routine, check out Hal Elrod's fantastic *The Miracle Morning*.

POWER IN THE EVENING

The "little brother" of the morning routine is the almost-as-important evening routine. Adopting an evening routine further cements the order you are imposing on your world by bookending your day with an additional set of positive and potent habits that compound the effect.

This is my current evening routine:

1. **Spend 10 minutes writing in a gratitude journal.**

Using a journal set aside exclusively for this practice, I open it to a fresh page and head it with the day's date. I then write the numbers one through five down the left margin and write down five things that I am grateful for that happened that day. It could be something positive that happened to me or a victory in something I've been working for, and it doesn't matter how small or insignificant it might seem.

2. **Enjoy 10 minutes of reflection.**

Using a quiet space where I will not be disturbed, I sit and reflect on the events of the day, paying particular attention to those I feel I could have handled better.

3. **Prepare for the following day.**

This is the most important part of the evening routine. I lay out my clothes for the next day as well as any items I'll require for my activities (paperwork, gym equipment, etc.). Then, using either a notepad or task management software, I list between one and three key things I need to complete the following day.

This serves two functions. First, by having everything ready to go and a clear plan of action, I am able to start my day with clarity and purpose and not waste precious energy deliberating about what I need to do or get distracted by trivial details. Second, listing what I want to achieve the next day allows my subconscious to begin working on those problems and challenges while I'm sleeping, ensuring that I have the greatest possible chance of successfully completing them when the time comes.

4. **Perform my sleep ritual.**

As outlined in chapter 13, this will ensure you have a great night's sleep, then wake up fresh and prepared to give your best.

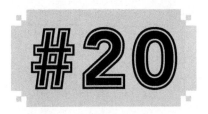

LOVE YOURSELF

— ★ ★ ★ —

> *Your greatest power is hidden in the last place you would ever want to look."*
>
> **—Nicholas Gregoriades**

A WEEK BEFORE this book was scheduled to be published, with very little warning, my wife left me for another man.

For some, this might have been just a sad and moderately challenging life event, but for me it was without question the most painful and difficult thing I have ever experienced.

I tried for a long time to find words to describe the effect it had on me, and the one I kept coming back to was *shattered*. My hopes, dreams, self-identity, and self-confidence were all completely shattered.

Up until that point, I had believed that my wife was my best friend and that we were happily married. I absolutely adored her and was totally dedicated to our future together. She and her needs were an integral part of my mission.

Sure, we had our challenges, as all couples do, but we had been through so much together, and each of us had sacrificed so much to make the relationship work that I really believed it was "ride or die" for both of us.

I didn't see it coming and I just wasn't prepared for it, so when I received the news, I went into a state of complete shock.

It took me on a journey into an abyss of confusion, despair, shame, guilt, and anger that was so dark and so deep, there were times I didn't think I was ever going to find my way out.

My mind tried so hard to make sense of it all that I couldn't sleep for weeks. I wept more over the next three months than I had in my whole life combined up until then. Physically, the stress on my system was so intense that my health began to fail and I developed a stomach ulcer.

I remember my rock-bottom moment very vividly. I was lying on the floor of my bathroom, crying while coughing up blood.

Even though my friends and family were there for me in spirit, I was separated from them not only geographically but by the ever-worsening circumstances surrounding COVID.

It was then that I understood *nobody was coming to save me*. I'd never, ever felt so alone, vulnerable, and disconnected from myself, others, and the world as a whole.

Today, four months later, as I write this, the fog of that experience is finally starting to clear. Despite all of the trauma, throughout it all I managed to maintain a focus on introspection and face it head-on.

As a younger man, I would have found some way to run away or distract myself from the excruciatingly uncomfortable feelings, but deep down I knew there was a lesson in what I was going through, one that I was determined to find and learn.

And eventually I did.

It's my current perspective that the Universe (or God, if you prefer) is always speaking to us and trying to guide us toward paths that are optimal for our health and growth. But sometimes we cannot hear it speak, and sometimes we hear it but refuse to listen. In these instances it's forced to "slap" us to wake us up.

In hindsight, I can now see that the failure of my marriage, something I had cherished and made every effort to succeed at, was a clarion call for me to wake up and realize that there was a crippling issue at play in my life that needed to be resolved:

I didn't fully love and accept myself.

Any token amounts of self-love and self-acceptance I'd had up until that point were contingent on external factors. The woman I was with, my appearance, how successful I was, my jiu jitsu black belt, etc.

And there were internal factors that had to be met, too: How "good" of a person I was. How much I believed I was helping others. How "conscious" I was. All of these things informed the way I felt about who I was at my core.

I can now identify the ways this chronic lack of self-love was mirrored in my marriage. For a long time, I had accepted so little—so little love, so little support, and so little affection. My wife had been checked out for months, and I hadn't been able to see it because I wanted so badly to believe in the fairytale.

I had loved her so totally and blindly that I had unknowingly placed her on a pedestal. I realized that all the positive traits I had projected onto her were elements of myself that I had failed to recognize and appreciate.

I remember speaking with a mentor of mine while I was at the depths of my confusion and trying to make sense of it all. "I just don't understand it," I said. "The day we got married, we looked into each other's eyes and made an oath. Didn't that mean anything to her?"

To which he answered, "Children cannot make oaths." It took me a long time to understand what he meant.

Almost without exception, human beings carry trauma from their childhoods, and that trauma will always seek to resolve itself. It does this by bringing people into our lives—especially romantic partners, who are perfectly positioned to trigger us. This invariably causes the trauma to be brought to the surface so that the emotions and energy tied to them can be felt, processed, and ultimately released.

We all have an inner child. This is an aspect of ourselves that is usually hidden, and it embodies not only childlike innocence and playfulness, but also all of the traumas mentioned above.

My parents are both deeply loving and wonderful people, but they are unfortunately, due to the family dynamics of their youth, emotionally stunted. I was raised by people who were still essentially children themselves.

Reflecting on this led to the challenging realization that what I was ultimately seeking in my romantic relationships was somebody who could be the adult this inner child had always desperately needed.

When it comes to our relationships with women, what men secretly crave is the same level of unconditional love that we received from our mothers. I'm sorry to be the one to have to tell you this, but this type of love is *exceedingly rare* in romantic relationships. The love a wife or girlfriend has for you is totally conditional. The conditions vary from person to person, but they absolutely exist. For us as men, this is an incredibly painful and disheartening truth to accept, but it's one that must be faced.

There is good news, though: even though you cannot get that type of love from a romantic partner or anyone else (besides your parents, perhaps), there is a far more dependable, eternal supply of unconditional love, and that's *you*. The only person who is able to give you the unwavering love you truly need is you.

I remember the exact moment I became a man. It wasn't when I got into a ring to fight another man. It wasn't when I had to make a difficult decision or sacrifice to provide for my family. It wasn't when I achieved success in the eyes of my father or the world.

It was when I stepped up and made a commitment to be there for my inner child. To unconditionally love, protect, and accept him regardless of the circumstances of my life. I chose to become the adult for *myself*.

I spent a long time deliberating on whether or not I should include this chapter in the book. I had concerns that it would make the reader feel that all the advice preceding it was invalid. I mean, how can you trust a guy claiming to have all these answers about manhood when he couldn't even keep his wife around? Some of my friends also commented that it broke the flow of the generally positive nature of the rest of the book.

I made a decision a long time ago that I would try to live a life of total authenticity. Hypocrisy and dishonesty are two characteristics I absolutely cannot tolerate, in myself or others. I realized that leaving out the impact and lessons of one the most powerful experiences of my life would have been inauthentic.

Ernest Hemingway once said, "The world breaks everyone, and afterward many are strong at the broken places."

When this event happened, it broke me. I can't pretend it didn't.

In the world of men, fragility and vulnerability are generally rejected and scorned. We're expected to be strong all the time and never show weakness. I see this so often on the jiu jitsu mat. But the truth is, we are all fragile and we are all vulnerable. You cannot armor yourself against life. It will always find a weak point in your defenses. Parts of it will be hard, and it's going to continually test you. And none of us knows what's around the corner—stuff you never saw coming will hit you when you least expect it.

But I can say that the guidance in this book will give you your best chance at getting up off the canvas when life inevitably knocks you down. It has been battle tested.

When I was broken and alone, I didn't lose myself in alcohol or porn. I meditated, took long walks in nature, and searched for the courage to look at the parts of me that were hurting. I drank ayahuasca and faced the darkness I found in myself. I did my best to maintain healthy routines and habits. But, most importantly, I kept listening to the soft, steady voice within that kept telling me, "Love yourself."

And that's why today I can look at the person in the mirror, see all of his flaws, failures, and insecurities, and still say he's the best man he's ever been.

IN CLOSING

ONE OF MY martial arts instructors, the legendary Roger Gracie, once said to me, "You can have anything you want in life as long as you are prepared to give what's required to get it."

If what you want is a life filled with joy, adventure, and success, then what's required of you is courage and action. Take the time and *do the work* required to become spiritually, mentally, and physically aligned, and you will live the life that you so richly deserve.

Thank you for reading this book and being dedicated to your own growth and evolution. It's men like you who lift the world up and make it a better place for everyone.

To close, I'd like to offer you the following blessing:

May the Great Spirit guide you, protect you, and give you peace beyond all understanding.

Your friend,
Nicholas Gregoriades

ABOUT THE AUTHOR

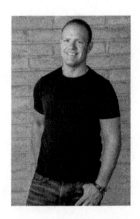

NIC GREGORIADES IS an entrepreneur, martial artist, psychonaut, and men's coach from Cape Town, South Africa.

In 2003 he moved to London, England, to earn his black belt in jiu jitsu. There he founded the popular martial arts community, the Jiu Jitsu Brotherhood. During that time he became the first person to be awarded a black belt by the legendary Roger Gracie and co-created the popular online show *London Real*.

In 2012, an encounter with the plant medicine ayahuasca in the Amazon profoundly affected his worldview and caused him to drastically change his life path. He spent the next five years traveling the world teaching jiu jitsu, studying yoga, and learning about the human experience.

He now lives in Los Angeles, California, where he runs his teaches and wellness business and works as a transformational coach for men looking to make profound life changes and reach their full potential.

WORK WITH NIC

MASTERMIND

> *Nic is amazing at gathering high-level people who feel safe to share openly about what's truly going on in their lives and who want to find the courage to make big changes. I'm so grateful to be a part of this group!"*
>
> **—Stephen Yeh, entrepreneur**

The hardest part of walking the path to success and fulfillment is doing it alone.

By becoming part of Nic's mastermind group, you'll gain access to a support network of men who are committed to the same thing you are: fulfilling their potential.

Find out more at: coachnicg.com/mastermind

RETREATS

> *My retreat with Nic was among the most transforma-tive experiences of my life. If you are looking for an abso-lutely safe environment to do the kind of deep self-explora-tion that you crave, I give my highest recommendation to Nicholas and his team."*
> **—Thomas Faustin-Huisking, entrepreneur**

Engage in a rejuvenating, powerful group experience to help you master your relationships with women, your family, your body, your career, and most importantly your Self.

Find out more at: <u>coachnicg.com/events</u>

1:1 COACHING

> *Nic and I have worked together to help me take owner-ship and experience liberation in key areas of my life."*
> **—Robert Upton, engineer**

Nic currently works one-to-one with a select group of men from around the world each year.

These individuals are *committed* to becoming the absolute best versions of themselves and value guidance and accountability.

Find out more at this link: <u>coachnicg.com/coaching</u>

FURTHER READING AND RESOURCES

BOOKS

Letting Go: The Pathway of Surrender by David R. Hawkins

No More Mister Nice Guy by Dr. Robert Glover

Necessary Endings by Dr. Henry Cloud

You Can Have It All by Arnold Patent

Unscripted by MJ DeMarco

The Oxygen Advantage by Patrick McKeown

Courage by OSHO

Deep Work by Cal Newport

The Testosterone Optimization Therapy Bible by Jay Campbell

PODCASTS

The Nicholas Gregoriades Show

Against the Rules with Michael Lewis

VIDEOS

Start with Why by Simon Sinek

Tidying Up with Marie Kondo

APPS

Sleep Cycle App

Insight Timer

Done Habit Tracking (iOS)

HabitBull (Android)

OTHER

Micropore Mouth Tape

Gradual Wake Alarm Clock

BDNF Nootropic Supplement

FOLLOW NIC

Follow Nic on Social Media

IG: @coach_nic_g

FB: facebook.com/coachnicg

You can sign up to stay in touch with Nic and his work, including his podcast, by visiting coachnicg.com

To contact nic directly email 1@coachnicg.com

The
Nicholas Gregoriades Show

The podcast for men seeking true health, wealth & fulfillment

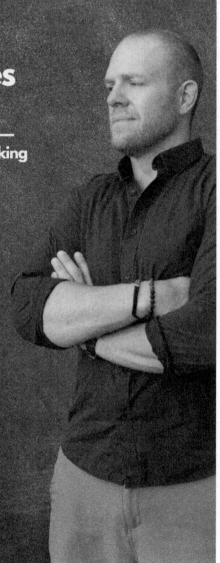

Available now in your favorite podcast app

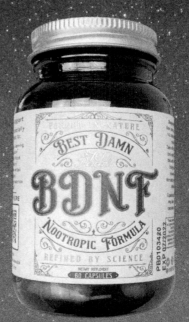

Printed in Great Britain
by Amazon

83310787R00088